Walid FEKI
Rahma GARGOURI
Rim KAMMOUN

Non-cystic fibrosis bronchial dilatation

Walid FEKI
Rahma GARGOURI
Rim KAMMOUN

Non-cystic fibrosis bronchial dilatation

Indicators of Severity

ScienciaScripts

Imprint

Cover image: www.ingimage.com

This book is a translation from the original published under ISBN 978-620-6-70492-8.

Publisher:
Sciencia Scripts
is a trademark of
Dodo Books Indian Ocean Ltd. and OmniScriptum S.R.L publishing group

120 High Road, East Finchley, London, N2 9ED, United Kingdom
Str. Armeneasca 28/1, office 1, Chisinau MD-2012, Republic of Moldova, Europe
Printed at: see last page
ISBN: 978-620-7-71184-0

Contents

1 Introduction

Bronchial dilatation (DDB) or bronchiectasis East a pathology respiratory chronic disabling characterized by an irreversible expansion of light small and medium bronchial caliber located between the [4th] and [8th] order of division (1).
Although the DDB has summer considered as underdiagnosed pathology , during the last five years its frequency has clearly increase due to the availability of high resolution CT scanning as well as epidemiological studies . In the United Kingdom , the prevalence of women increased from 350.5 per 100,000 inhabitants in 2004 to 566.1 in 2013 and that of men from 301.2 per 100,000 inhabitants in 2004 to 485.5 per 100,000 inhabitants in 2013 (2). The data global confirm the important morbidity and health care burden associated with this disorder particularly in people socio- economically disadvantaged . According to a recent review of the literature (3) the cost of illness has summer mainly due to hospitalizations among patients having a history of repeated exacerbations .
Recurrent infections are responsible of attacks tissue and inflammation leading to the production of excess mucus associated with an alteration of the mucociliary carpet . Subsequently, a vicious COLE cycle of tissue destruction and superinfections bronchial go be triggered (4) at the origin of occurrence exacerbations and consequently decline in function respiratory (5.6).
To properly take care of these patients, the clinician must first :
- Identify patients very symptomatic , at risk of exacerbations severe and those whose function respiratory collapsed . These sick are the target of a socket in multidisciplinary responsibility and a therapeutic relatively reinforced . Contrary , patients at light risk have a socket simpler support not requiring monitoring specializes .

Two severity scores specific to DDB have summer elaborate whose aim is to better perceive the impact of the illness and thus guide the treatment in therapeutic charge of the clinician : bronchiectasis severity index (BSI) (7) and FACED score (8.9).
Each of the two scores allocates points intended for age , value in percentage of maximum expiry volume in a second (FEV), the presence of a colonization by Pseudomonas Aeruginosa, the extension radiological and stage of dyspnea according to the MRC scale . The BSI score assigns in addition, points for body mass index (BMI), frequency of exacerbations, notion of hospitalization , colonization by a bacterium other than Pseudomonas Aeruginosa. Subsequently , the calculation of the scores will arrive at a classification of patients into three risk groups : mild , moderate and high .
The BSI score has summer established following a large study in Edinburgh in United Kingdom , subsequently validated by 4 cohorts international . As for the FACED score, it was established during of a Spanish retrospective study and

evaluated independently in a single- center cohort in Kingdom Uni.The FACED score was developed specifically for mortality prediction while the BSI score allows a prediction of mortality , severe exacerbations as well as the frequency of exacerbations and allows an estimate of quality of life (10,11,12,13).
Several settings can influence these two scores , notably factors specific to each population.
No study has checked the applicability of these 2 severity scores and has no evaluates the best score for our population.
The aim of our study is to research a possible correlation that could exist between the different severity parameters as well as the BSI and FACED score scores and to therefore be able to choose the best score for our population.

2 Patients and Methods

1. Type of study

It 's about of a comparative, single- center study (Pneumology department of the Hedi Chaker University Hospital of Sfax), covering the period going from 1st January 2009 until December 31, 2018.

2. Study population

2.1.Criteria of inclusion

- Age > 16 years
- Dilation of the bronchi confirmed by chest scan

2.2.Non-inclusion criteria

Patients with cystic fibrosis .

Dilation of the bronchi accompanying other pathologies including pulmonary fibrosis and bronchopulmonary cancer .

3. Data collection

We have consults the medical records of selected patients and collects some number of data clinical , para- clinical and therapeutic .

file analysis grid has summer established for each patient in order to to obtain data Also homogeneous as possible (Appendix 1).

Elements of the interrogation

Age

Sex

Personal history

Family history of neoplasia

Lifestyle habits

The signs functional respiratory , extra respiratory and general .

Hemoptysis has summer sought in all patients. Gravity has summer evaluated in function of the objective bleeding volume , the underlying terrain (insufficiency underlying respiratory system) and the impact on the state respiratory and hemodynamic .

3.1.. Clinical examination data

- patient's general condition (World Health Organization performance status index)
- The state respiratory :

o Presence of bronchial rales , crackling rales see wheezing during auscultation pulmonary witnesses of congestion bronchial .

o A digital clubbing that can translate a insufficiency evolutionary respiratory .

Extra respiratory signs : signs of insufficiency right heart , sinusitis which can to have a value in orientation diagnostic .

3.2.. Additional tests

3.2.1. Imaging

Chest x-ray

She is often pathological and allows to objectify two types of anomalies .

Direct anomalies

S Clarites tubular : correspond to visibility spontaneous wall bronchial thickened through the non-condensed parenchyma .

S Clartes annular (areolar images): Same thing seen sectional

S Tubulated opacities in " V " or in " Y " : correspond to bronchi full oriented according to the bronchial axis . Their translations are the mucoid impactions with para- hilar distribution and the bronchocele instead lobar .

S Rosette appearance or in "pseudo-honeycomb " : this is the translation of bronchiectasis cylindrical Or varicose veins , juxtaposed one after the other against others and views in cross sections .

S Multi- cavitary appearance within which can exist levels liquidians . It is the translation radiology of bronchiectasis saccular Or cystic .

Indirect anomalies

S Images of atelectasis and collapse United or multi- lobar

Chest scan

chest scanner had a great contribution to our study. He was request in fine, millimetric sections and allowed of :

- Put evidence of bronchial dilation in front one of the following situations :

S the intra- bronchial diameter East greater than that of the satellite artery

S the bronchi are visualized at the level of the outer 1/3 of the parenchyma pulmonary

S absence of progressive reduction in caliber bronchial , as we moves away from the hilae .

- Determine the type of bronchial dilatation : cylindrical , moniliform , cystic according to Reid's classification.
- Assess the extent of the DDB
- Specify any possible complications.

3.2.2. Spirometry

Spirometry made it possible to measure the function respiratory tract of patients and therefore determine the type of abnormality functional respiratory as well as its degree of severity . Spirometry was not carried out in patients having a medical contraindication .

3.2.3. Cytobacteriological examination of sputum

The exam cytobacteriological analysis of sputum made it possible to detect the type of infection or colonization which can be an indirect sign of severity . Colonization bacterial was defined following the recommendations Spanish (14) by the presence of the same germ on 2 sputum samples during the year previous and at least 3 months old interval .

3.3.Severity scores

Charlson comorbidity index (CCI)

This score has summer used in order to to study comorbidities and predict short- and long- term survival (15). This score is consists of 19 categories of comorbidities (Appendix 2). Each disease has a different weighting according to the strength of its association with mortality after a year. The total CCI score is calculated in adding the weights associated with each comorbid disorder presented by the patient . Higher scores indicate more severe disorders and, consequently, a poorer prognosis .

The BSI score

This score includes 9 variables (Appendix 3). The total score corresponds to the sum of the scores for each variable and varies between 0 and 26 points. Depending on the total score, patients will be classified into 3 groups : low BSI score (0-4 points), intermediate BSI score (5-8 points), high BSI score (> 9).

The FACED score

This score includes 5 dichotomous variables (Appendix 4). The total score corresponds to the sum of the scores for each variable and varies between 0 and 7 points.

It allows DDB to be classified into 3 risk groups : mild DDB (0-2 points), moderate (3-4 points) and severe (5-7 points).

Estimation of quality of life

***Le St Georges Respiratory Questionnaire (SGRQ)**

This score has summer valid for certain respiratory pathologies such as bronchopneumopathy chronic obstructive pulmonary disease (COPD) and asthma . He was valid during the DDB and translated in several languages (16,17). The SGRQ includes 50 items distributed in 3 dimensions : symptoms , activity and impact on activity professional , daily life and impact emotional . A score varying from 0 to 100 will be assigned for each dimension, as well as the total score. (Appendix 5)

***Echelle HAD (Hospital Anxiety And Depression scale)**

It is a scale that allows the screening of anxiety and depressive disorders . It includes 14 items rated from 0 to 3. Seven questions relate to anxiety (total A) and seven others to the depressive dimension (total D), allowing Thus obtaining 2 scores. For each dimension, a score ranging from 0 to 7 means an absence of symptoms , between 8 and 10 means a symptomatology doubtful and from 11 means a symptomatology certain . If we considered the two dimensions together, a higher score or equal to 15 is a score in favoring anxiety - depressive disorders . (Appendix 6)

3.4.Therapeutics used

The type of treatment has summer evaluated by the doctor investigator . More illness was severe, the more treatment was intense.

3.5.Evolution and survival

For survival and evolution , we are refer to patient files When they contained information on evolution . For patients lost to follow-up , we have try to contact them or contact their parents by mail or telephone.

4. Statistic study

The data have summer entered and analyzed using SPSS II version 20 software . The values digital have summer expressed in average more or less standard - deviation . The association between qualitative variables East calculated by the Chi2 test corrected by Fisher for small numbers . Comparisons between quantitative variables have summer done with the Student's T test. The meaning is acquired for a $p < 0.05$ for all statistical tests .

3 Results

1. Study of the global population

1.1.Epidemiology

1.1.1. Impact

We have collects 110 cases . Characteristics overall number of patients followed have summer summarized in Table II. To calculate severity scores and during the whole part of the study prognosis , we have excluded 8 patients not having had a spirometry due to non - cooperation .

Sex

The population has summer characterized by a sex ratio of 1.4 , i.e. 64 men (58%) and 46 women (42%) (Figure 1).

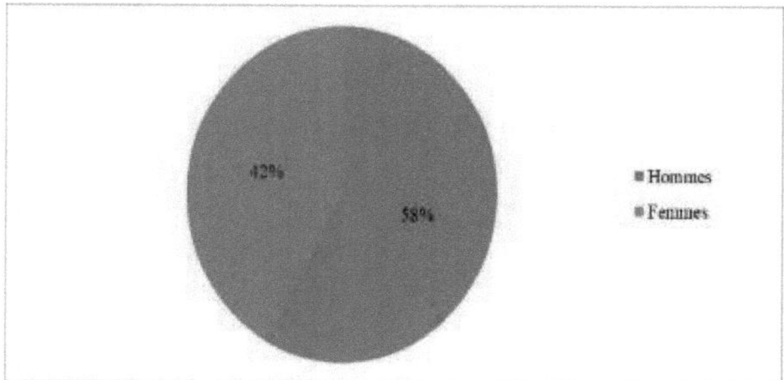

Figure 1 : Distribution of patients by gender

1.1.2. Age

Age The average patient age was 60 years with extremes ranging from 16 to 90 years and a peak frequency in the age group over 70 years . (Figure 2)

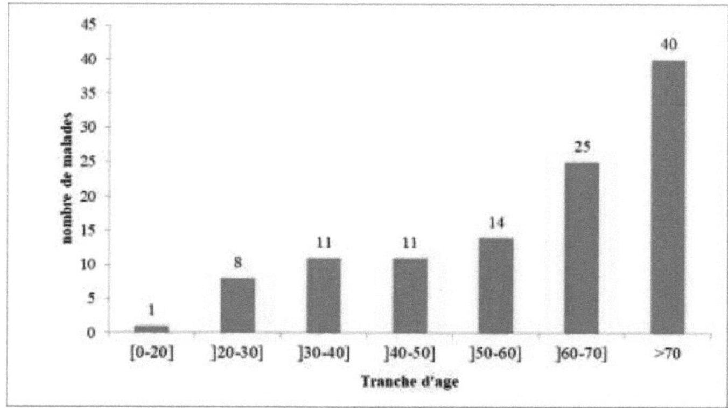

Figure 2: Distribution of patients according to age group

1.1.3. Habits

1.1.3.1. Smoking

We have collects 50 smoking patients assets among our population with a male predominance of 95%. The number of packets year AVERAGE has summer of 26 AP. The withdrawal smoking was obtained for 24 patients .

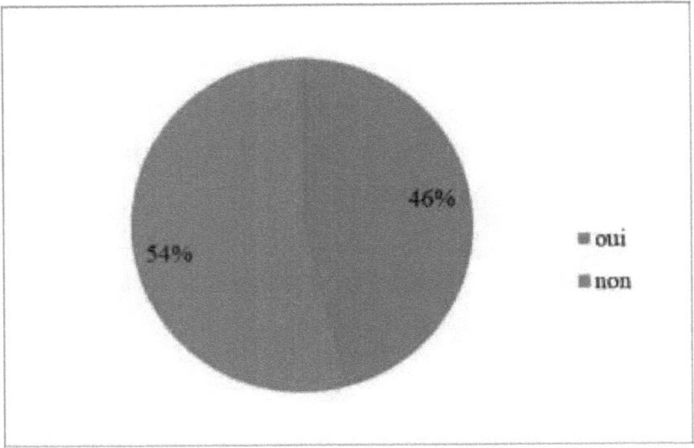

Figure 3: Percentage of smoking in the population

1.1.3.2. Alcoholism

Among our population we have has 3 patients alcoholics 2 of whom were at the stage of liver cirrhosis .

1.1.4. Personal history

Personal medical history summer found in 92 patients, or 84% of cases . Gastroesophageal reflux disease (GERD) and hypertension arterial have been dominant. Body mass index has summer calculated for all patients , the average CMI was 23.39 with extremes ranging from 13 to 38.

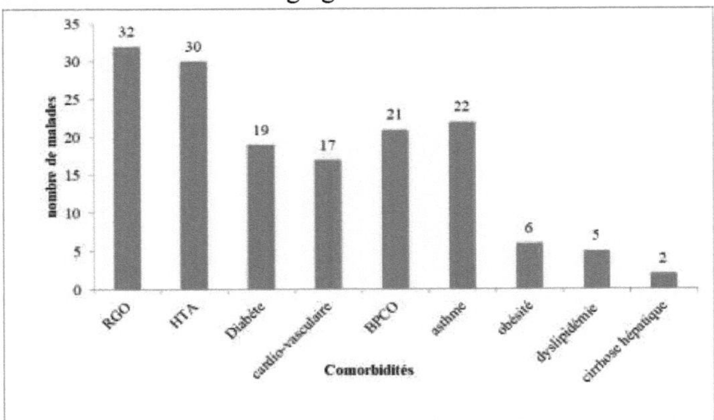

Figure 4: Distribution of patients' personal medical history

The Charlson score (CCI) has summer calculated for all patients . Thirteen patients have had a CCI equal to 0, the majority of patients have had a score between 1 and 4 (66%) (Figure 5).

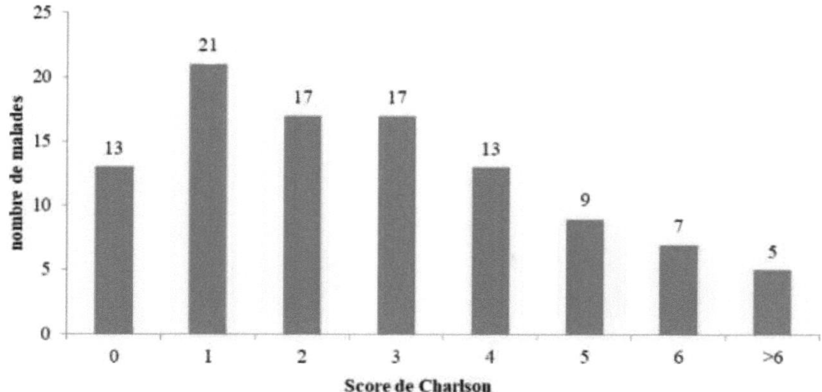

Figure 5: Distribution of patients according to the Charlson score

1.1.5. Socio- economic level

We have divided the population into 3 categories according to the level socio-economic status of patients based on particularly on the profession, the city origin and living conditions.

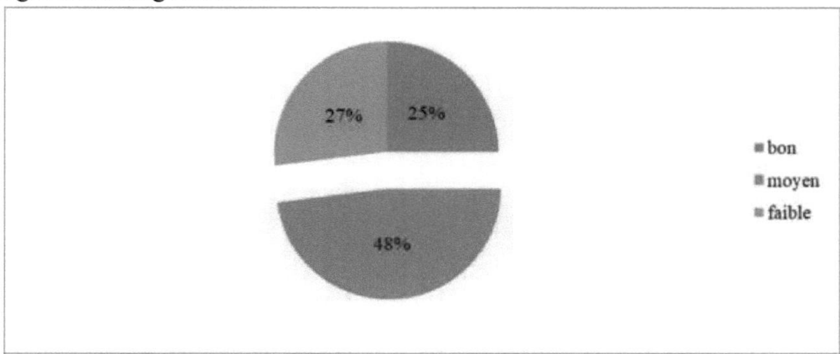

Figure 6: Distribution of patients according to level socioeconomic

1.2.Clinical study

Functional signs respiratory

By questioning the patients, we looked for the main symptoms respiratory tract during DDB : dyspnea stress , hemoptysis and bronchorrhea morning . Others signs clinics have been researched such as cough chronic particularly productive, pain thoracic and recurrent lower respiratory infections (Figure 7).

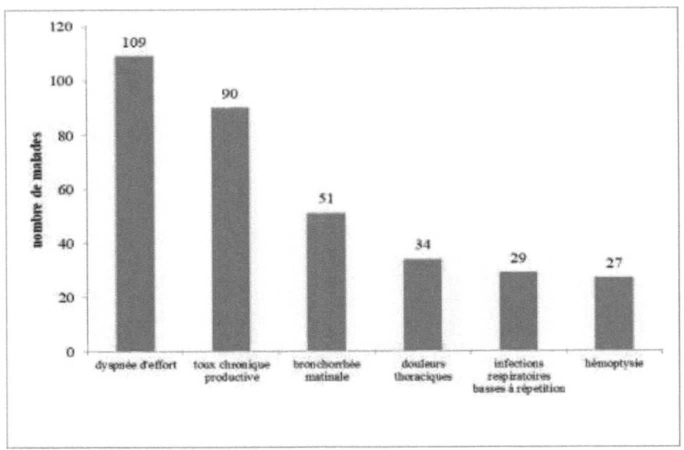

Figure 7 : Symptoms during DDB

Dyspnea effort :

Dyspnea of effort represented the sign most common clinic . Using the MRC classification, we find that the majority of our population has been at stage 3. (Figure 8)

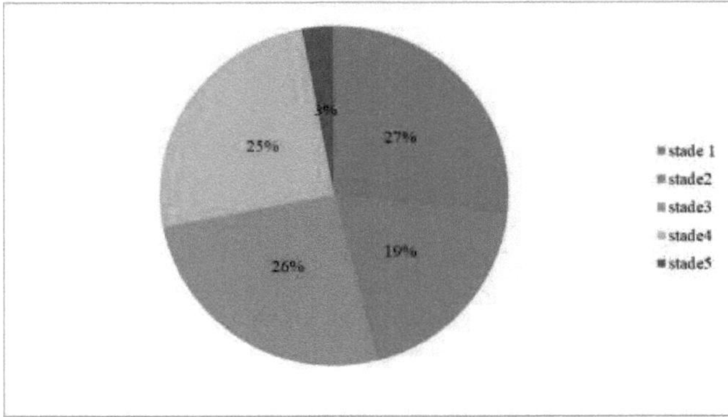

Figure 8: Distribution of patients depending on dyspnea of effort

Cough productive:

Concerning productive cough, we noted that the color of sputum, apart from episodes of exacerbations , summer very variable. (Figure 9)

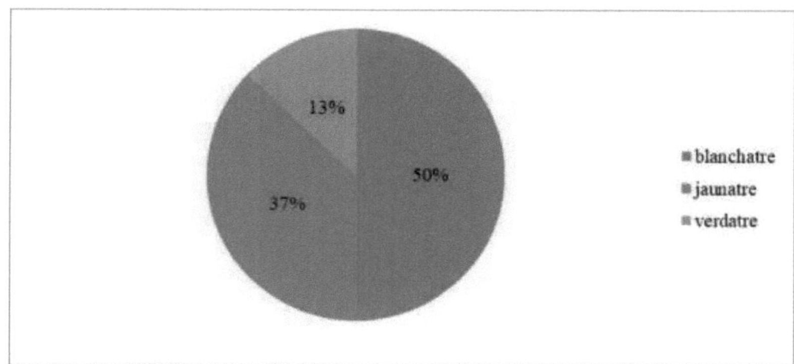

Figure 9: The color of sputum in patients outside of exacerbations

Hemoptysis :

In front of all hemoptysis , we looked for signs of severity with an assessment of abundance . Severe hemoptysis with recourse to a embolization in emergency summer diagnosed in 2 patients . Recurrence of hemoptysis concerned 16 cases . examination :

Outside of pushes infectious , physical examination has was normal in 85% of cases . Upstairs thoracic , abnormalities on auscultation pulmonary have was dominated by bronchial rales snoring . A digital clubbing has was observed in 15 patients more readily in extensive and old forms .

1.3.Paraclinical study

1.3.1 Imaging thoracic

1.3.1.1 Radiography standard thoracic

A radiograph thoracic has summer practiced in all patients returning pathological in 95% of cases . We looked for direct anomalies especially the clarity tubular (30%), clear annular (25%) and multi- cavitary images (45%). (Figure 10)

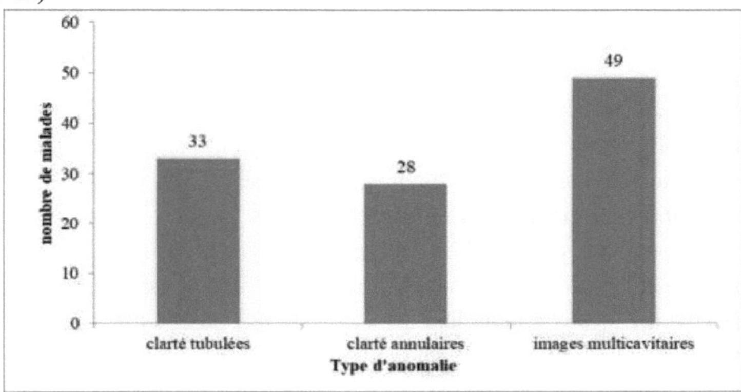

Figure 10: Description of abnormalities on chest x-ray

We have studied using chest CT the topography as well as the type of lesions. We noted the predominance of lesions at the level of 2 lobes (38%). The average of affected lobes has was 3.27.

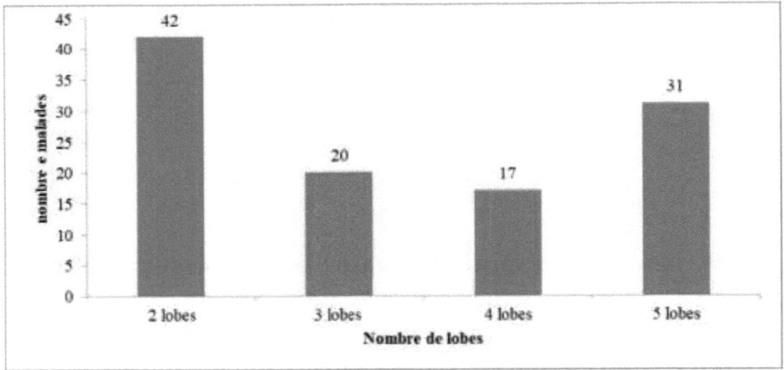

Figure 11: The number of affected lobes in our population

Shapes cylindrical were the most present in our population followed by forms cystic Then moniliform (Figure 12). Associations between the *3* types have summer observed in 51.9% of cases . Emphysema has was present in 30.4% of cases .

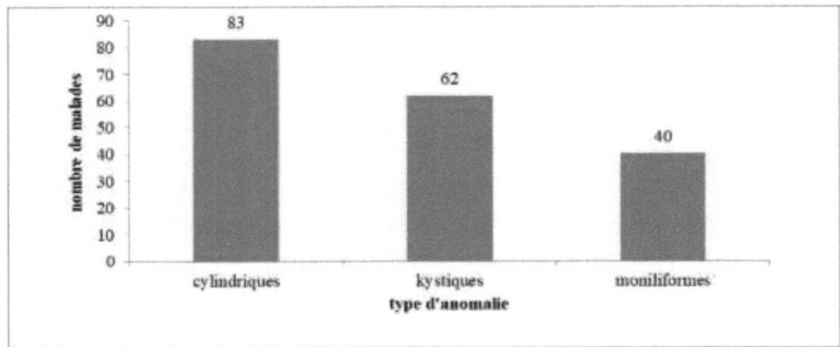

Figure 12: Types of lesions on chest CT

Others affected associates such as lymphadenopathy mediastino-hilar were frequent (32%). Their topography mediastinal has summer predominant (91%). A pleurisy associate has summer diagnosed in 4 cases .

1.3.2 Cytobacteriological examination of sputum

An ECBC has been practiced in all patients . Twenty -four patients have summer infected with Pseudomonas Aeruginosa , 5 of which were colonized . Likewise, twenty -two patients had a history of secondary infection by a germ other than pyocyanic but without being colonized by these germs .

Functional exploration respiratory

The value average FEV1 was 52 % with extremes ranging from 17% to 93 %.

We have split our population in 4 groups according to the value in percentage of FEV1 (Table 1). A ventilatory disorder obstructive has summer found in 49 cases and the restrictive disorder of fagon less in 30 cases .

Table I: Distribution of patients according to FEV1

Band	FEV1	(not)	%
light	> 80	8	7
Moderate	50-80	53	48
Severe	30-49	34	31
very severe	<30	15	14
Total		**110**	

Table II: Features general characteristics of patients in our population

Patient characteristics	
Sex	46? ; 64 days
Average age (year)	60
BMI (average)	23.39
Dyspnea MRC (median)	3
FEV (%)	52%
Colonization by Pseudomonas Aeruginosa	5
Colonization by others germs	0
Number of lobes affected (average)	3
Exacerbation the year previous (average)	2
Hospitalization in the previous 2 years (average)	1.42

1.3.4 Etiologies of DDB

Investigation etiological has summer requested for all patients . It has been noted that DDB of unknown origin (idiopathic) has summer majority representing 65% of cases .

The etiologies have summer characterized by their variability . Tuberculosis pulmonary has summer diagnosed in 21 patients (19%), secondary DDB has a pneumopathy severe infectious disease during childhood have summer found in 10 patients (9%). Likewise, a system disease or one vasculitis has summer diagnosed in 8 cases , we cite for example polyarthritis rheumatoid (n=5), Gougerot Sjogren syndrome (n=2) and Wegener's disease (n=1).

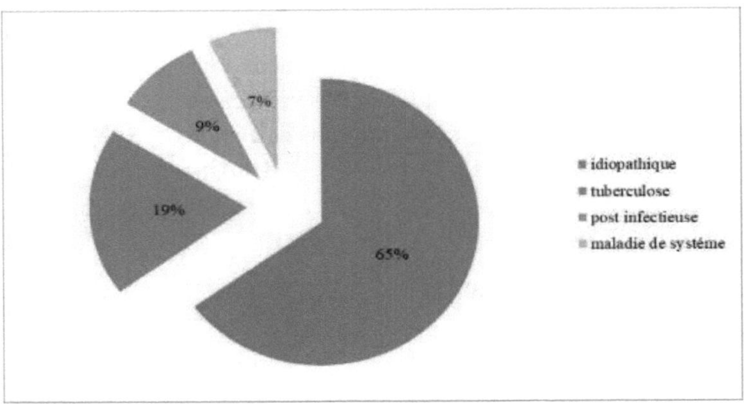

Figure 13: Etiologies of DDB

1.3.5 DDB processing

Treatment during DDB has summer characterize by the variability of prescription and depends enormously on the signs patient clinics . We have illustrates the different medications used during DDB in Figure 14 .

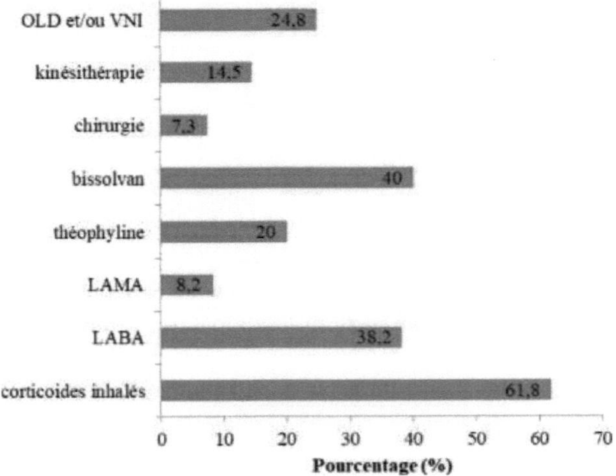

Figure 14 : Medications used during DDB

1.4 Prognostic study

We have excluded in this part 8 sick not having had a spirometry (non-cooperating), thus not allowing the calculation of severity scores . The total number of patients in this part will be like this reduced to 102 cases .

1.4.1 Mortality

1.4.1.1 Mortality rate

Twenty -one patients were died when carrying out the study . Death rate was thus 20.6%.

1.4.1.2 Factors predictions :

1.4.1.2.1 Age:

The average age among patients died has was 69±17.6 years and in survivors 57.6±17.59 years with a statistically significant difference (p=0.009).

Mortality increases with age , it goes from 2% for patients aged under 40 to 4.9% between 40 and 65 years and 13.7% for patients over 65 years old. The difference is not statistically significant.

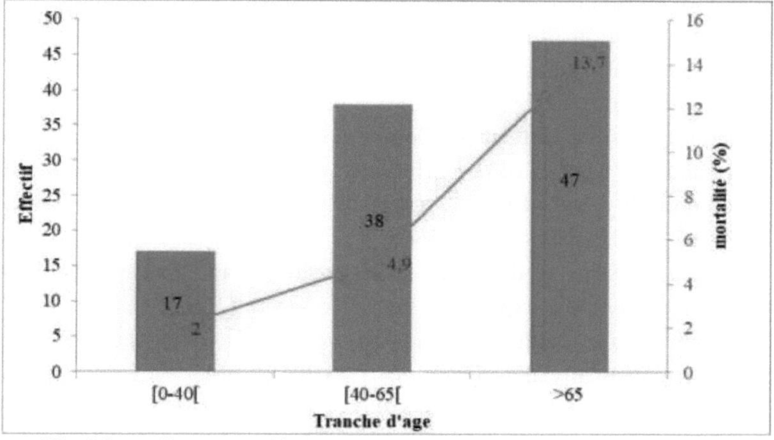

Figure 15 : Mortality according to age group

Table III: Cross- tabulation deaths and age group

Age group (years)	Death		Total
	NOT	%	
0-40	2	2	17
41-65	5	4.9	38
>65	14	13.7	47
total	21	20.6	**102**

1.4.1.2.2 Gender

The distribution of deaths according to sex showed a predominance of sex masculine . In fact , fifteen sex deaths male or 25.9% have summer postpone against 6 of sex feminine i.e. 13.6% with a statistically insignificant difference (p=0.13).

Table IV: Distribution of deaths in gender function

Décès	Sexe		Total
	Femme	Homme	
Non	38	43	81
Oui	6	15	21
%	13,6	25,9	-
Total	44	58	**102**

1.4.1.2.3 Socio- economic level

Among our population , most patients deceased (n=21) had a good to average level socio-economic with a statistically significant link (p=0.01).

1.4.1.2.4 Comorbidities

We looked for possible correlations between, on the one hand, mortality and, on the other hand, the number of comorbidities , the Charlson score and finally the type of comorbidity . We found a statistically significant relationship between mortality and Charlson score (p=0.004).

The ill having a history of diabetes , hypertension, heart disease ischemic have summer statistically more exposed to the risk of death (Table V).

Mortality has summer high in patients having a BMI lower than 18 reaching 47.1% with a statistically significant link (p=0.001) (Table VI).

Table V: Distribution of deaths according to comorbidities

	Number of patients	**Death**		**p-value**
		NOT	%	0.034
Diabetes	18	7	38.8	
HT	28	1242.9		0.001
Heart disease ischemic	10	5	50	0.015
COPD	21	7	33.3	0.1
Asthma	22	2	9.1	0.13
Reflux	32	4	12.5	0.17
Obesity	5	0	0	0.24
Measles	0	0	0	-

Table VI: Distribution of deaths according to weight status

Death	**Weight status**										**Total**
	<18		18-24		25-29		30-40		>40		-
	not	%	not	%	not	%	not	%	not	%	

No	9	52.9	26	68.4	38	97.4	7	100	1	100	81
Yes	8	47.1	12	31.6	1	2.6	0	0	0	0	21
Total	**17**		**38**		**39**		**7**		**1**		**102**

1.4.1.2.5 Quality of life

The St Georges questionnaire could not be carried out in patients died what has us stop to estimate the quality of life in this particular case .

1.4.1.2.6 Tobacco

Twelve death have were active cigarette smokers . The number of packets year AVERAGE has summer 26 AP. The connection was not statistically significant (p=0.25).

1.4.1.2.7 Hemoptysis

Five deaths have summer accounts among the sick presenting a hemoptysis . The connection was not statistically significant (p= 0.51). The abundance of hemoptysis has summer weak for the sick deaths (p= 0.28). The recurrence of hemoptysis in these sick has summer observed in 2 cases (p=0.21).

1.4.1.2.8 Number of exacerbations

The number of exacerbation AVERAGE was 2 with extremes of 1 to 12 exacerbations/year. We noted a peak in deaths at 9 coinciding with patients having 2 exacerbations/year. The connection has summer statistically significant (p=0.034) (Figure 16)

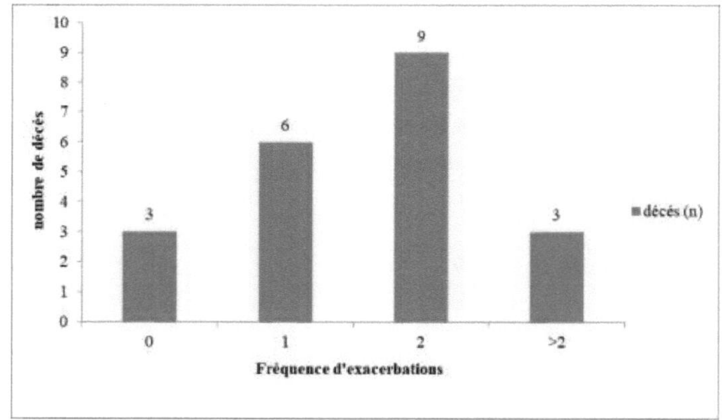

Figure 16: Distribution of deaths according to the frequency of exacerbations

1.4.1.2.9 Number of hospitalizations

The number AVERAGE hospitalization was 1.42 during the 2 years previous ones . We have seen a spike in morality coinciding with the sick having a history of hospitalization in the previous 2 years . The connection has summer statistically significant (p=0.004). None case of death n / A was noted in patients who had not been hospitalized within the past two years .

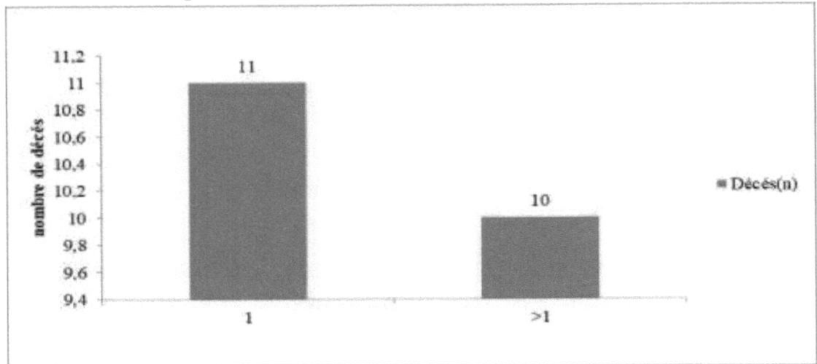

Figure 17: Distribution of deaths according to the frequency of hospitalization

1.4.1.2.10 Infection

The presence of a history of superinfection with Pseudomonas has was observed in 19 patients of which 2 have summer died . No correlation has summer established with mortality in our population. (p=0.49)

Colonization by Pseudomonas affected 4 patients of which only 1 died . No correlation has summer established with mortality . (p=0.82)

We are looking for a possible superinfection by germs other than Pseudomonas. Likewise, no statistical link with mortality was found . We have illustrates the results of the different germs in the attached table. Colonization by one of these germs was not found in our series to study its relationship with mortality .

Table VII: The correlation between death and the different objective microorganisms at ECBC

Germ	not	Death		P
		not%		
Pseudomonas Aeruginosa	19	211		0.49
Aspergillosis	3	0	0	0.57
Branhamella catarrhalis	5	240		0.27
Candida albicans	2	0	0	0,46
E.Coli	1	0	0	0,60
Haemophilus Influenzae	4	125		0,82
Pneumocoque	3	133		0,57
Kleibsielle pneumoniae	1	0	0	0,6
Acinetobacter Baumani	1	0	0	0,60
Serratia Marcosuras	2	150		0.29

1.4.1.2.11 The function respiratory

We are looking for a possible relationship between the percentage of FEV1

according to the 4 groups and survival in our population. In fact , we have got the results following : we did not find any deaths in the mild group unlike the others groups among which 6, 10 and 5 deaths have summer respectively found in groups moderate , severe and very severe (p=0.034).
An analysis of mortality according to the Kaplan and Meier survival curves did not show a statistically significant difference between the 4 groups (p=0.71).

1.4.1.2.12 DDB type

We have studies the relationship between the 3 types of DDB with mortality (while knowing that they can be associated). The number of deaths was not significantly different depending on the type of DDB and also depending on the presence or absence of emphysema and lymphadenopathy hilars Or mediastinales . In fact , the number of deaths reached respectively 20%, 19% and 19% respectively for the cylindrical , cystic and moniliform types (table VIII).

Table VIII: Distribution of deaths in function of radiological abnormalities on chest CT

Kind	not	Death		P
		not	%	
Cylindrical	75		1520	0.86
Moniliform	37	7	19	0.89
Cystic	59		1119	0.77
Associations	53	9	17	0.48
Emphysema	31	8	26	0.38
Adenopathy mediastinal / hilar	35	7	20	0.91

1.4.1.2.13 Etiology

The etiologies that we found have summer characterized by their variability . Tuberculosis pulmonary has summer diagnosed in 19 patients including 4 patients died or 21.1%. A secondary DDB has a pneumopathy severe infectious disease during childhood summer found in 9 patients of which only 1 died . Likewise, a system disease has summer diagnosed for 7 patients including 2 deaths and a single case of vasculitis (Wegener) without objective death .
No statistical relationship n / A summer established between the different etiologies and mortality (Table IX)

Table IX: Distribution of deaths in function of the etiology of DDB

Etiology	NOT	Death		P
		not	%	
Tuberculosis	19	4	21.1	0.95

Post- infectious	9	1	11.1	0.46
System disease	7	2	28.6	0.58
Idiopathic	67		1420.9	0.91
Total	102		2120.6	

1.4.1.2.14 Treatment

We do not have an objective relationship between mortality and treatment except for the use of Bromhexine (p=0.034).

Table X : Mortality in treatment function

Medicine	**NOT**	**Death**		**P**
		not	%	
Inhaled corticosteroids	64	13	61.9	0.93
LAMA	8	2	9.5	0.75
OVER THERE	40	8	38.1	0.91
Theophyline	21	4	19	0.85
Bromhexine	40	4	19	0.034
Surgery	8	2	25	0.75
OLD and/ or NAV	25	7	28	0.24
Physiotherapy respiratory	14	2	14	0.53

Severity scores

BSI and FACED scores

We have studies the variables defining the FACED and the BSI score. The distribution of patients by variable according to each score has summer illustrated in tables 9 and 10.

We then studied the characteristics of the patients in each of the 3 risk groups for each score .We have find a difference in the distribution of patients depending on the score used .

1.4.2.1 FACED score

Based on the FACED score the results have summer as follows: the “mild” group included 32 patients (31.4%), “ moderate ” group 48 patients (47%) and group “ severe ” 22 patients (21.6%).

Table XI: The FACED score

Variable	**Sample (n=102)**	
	not	%
FEV1		
<50%	56	55

>50%	46	45
Age (year)		
>70	33	32
<70	69	68
Colonization by Pseudomonas		
Aeruginosa	98	96
No	4	4
Yes		
Radiological extension		
>2 lobes	102	100
<2 lobes	0	0
Dyspnee- mMRC		
> II (III et IV)	47	46
< II (0- II)	55	54

1.4.2.2 BSI score

The BSI score made it possible to classify patients in band " mild " including 22 patients (21.6%), " moderate" » corresponding to 21 patients (20.6%) and severe to 59 patients (57.8%).

Table XII: The BSI score

Variable	**Sample (n=102)**	
	NOT	%
Age (year) <50	46	45
50-69	31	30
70-79	14	14
>80	11	11
Body mass index (BMI) <18.5	9	9
>18.5	93	91
FEV(%)		
>80%	12	12
50-80%	45	44
30-49%	31	30
<30%	14	14
Hospitalizations in the previous 2 years no	31	30
Yes	71	70
Exacerbations during the year previous 0-2	72	71
>3	30	29
Dyspnea - CKD 1-3	74	73
4	26	25
5	2	2
Colonization by Pseudomonas Aeruginosa no	98	96
Yes	4	4
Colonization by another microorganism no	102	100
Yes	0	0
Radiological extension (> 3 lobes and/ or cystic DDB) no	61	59

Yes	41	41

1.4.2.3 Link between BSI and FACED scores

bivariate study showed a statistically significant link between the BSI and the FACED scores (Pearson test, p<0.0001).

Table XIII: Classification of patients by FACED and BSI scores

BSI	FACED			
	Light	**moderate**	**Severe**	**Total**
Light	14 (43.8%)	5 (104%)	3 (13.6%)	22 (21.6%)
Moderate	6 (18.8%)	14 (29.2%)	1 (4.5%)	21 (20.6%)
Severe	12 (37.5%)	29 (60.4%)	18 (81.8%)	59 (57.8%)
Total	32 (31.4%)	48 (47.1%)	22 (21.6%)	102 (100%)

Severity scores and mortality

The BSI score has was more sensitive than the FACED score for predicting mortality with a greater area under the curve (AUC) (0.77 versus 0.67) and a more significant p value (p<0.0001).

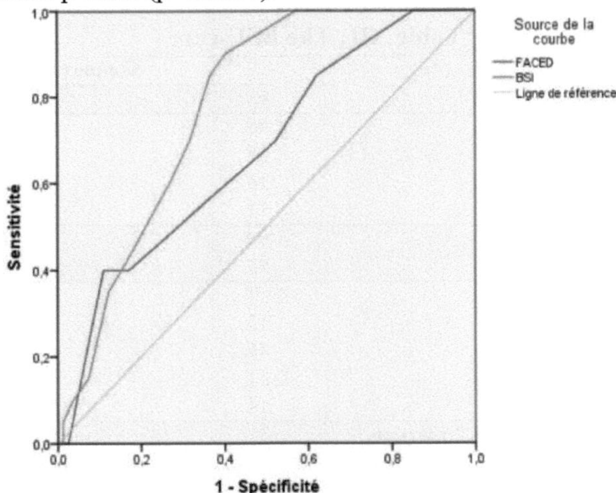

Figure 18: ROC curve : Mortality according to FACED and BSI scores

Severity scores and prediction of hospitalizations

The ill hospitalized a times during the previous two years are mainly those in the severe and moderate group respectively for the BSI and FACED score and with a superiority for the BSI since it brings together 24 patients versus 18 for FACED. If we are interested in the sick hospitalized more than one times the previous two years we found 34 patients classified as severe BSI versus 18 moderate FACED patients . (table XIV)

The BSI score has was more sensitive than the FACED score for predicting hospitalizations with a greater AUC (0.95 versus 0.69) and a more significant p value (p<0.0001).

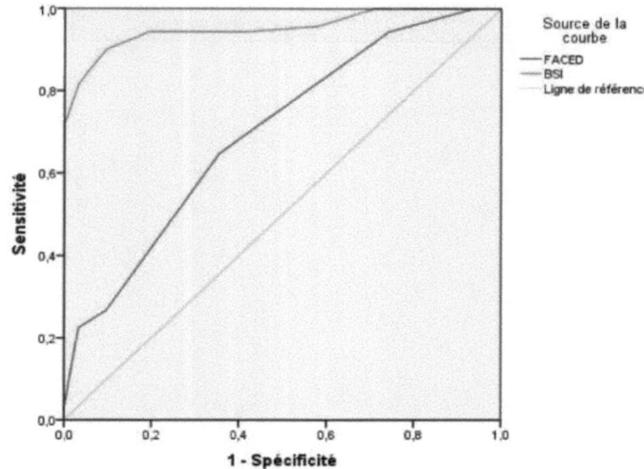

Figure 19: ROC curve : Hospitalizations according to FACED and BSI scores

Table XIV: Distribution of hospitalizations in function of the severity score

	Hospitalization n=1			Hospitalization n >1		
	Light	Moderate	Severe	Light	Moderate	Severe
BSI	4	7	24	0	2	34
FACED	10	18	7	6	18	12

Severity scores and prediction of exacerbations

Patients who have had 2 exacerbations per year former are mainly those in the severe and moderate group respectively for the BSI and FACED score (11 patients versus 13 respectively). More frequent exacerbations beyond 2 have were objective in patients classified as severe by the BSI score numbering 28 but also in the group moderate via FACED in 15 patients . (Table XV).

The difference between the two scores was not significant with an AUC of around 0.65 and 0.64 respectively for the FACED and the BSI scores and a similar p- value (p=0.02). These results show that the 2 scores are can sensitive in the prediction of exacerbations since their corresponding AUCs do not exceed 0.7.

Table XV: The distribution of exacerbations in depending on the score of Gravite

Exacerbation n=2 Exacerbation n >2

	Light	Moderate	Severe	Light	Moderate	Severe [1]
BSI	4	6	11	1	1	28
FACED	5	13	3	8	15	7

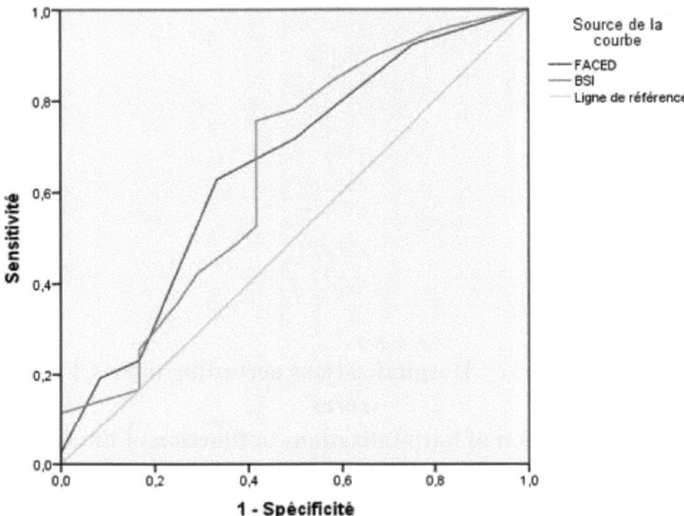

Figure 20: ROC curve : exacerbations according to FACED and BSI

Severity scores and survival

The distribution of deaths within the risk groups showed their predominance in the severe group for BSI where the majority of patients are found . deaths (20 patients) with only one patient belonging to the group moderate , unlike the FACED score, where we find the distribution of deaths like the following : 3 in the light group (10%), 10 in the group moderate (21%) and 8 in the severe group (36%). (Table XVI)

Table XVI: The number of deaths in function of the severity score

	Topics	**Deaths**	
		N	N %
BSI			
Light	22	0	0
Moderate	21	1	5
Severe	59	20	34
FACED			
Light	32	3	10
Moderate	48	10	21

Severe	22	8	36

We have constructs the ten- year survival curves of Kaplein and Meyer according to the FACED and BSI scores. The curves have summer different in function of the severity score used .

For the BSI score : The survival curve shows a mortality important and early in the severe group . Mortality in the mild and moderate groups is not significant, the survival curve in this case East horizontal .

For the FACED score : mortality mainly reaches groups moderate and severe with decreasing survival curve quickly and especially for the severe group .

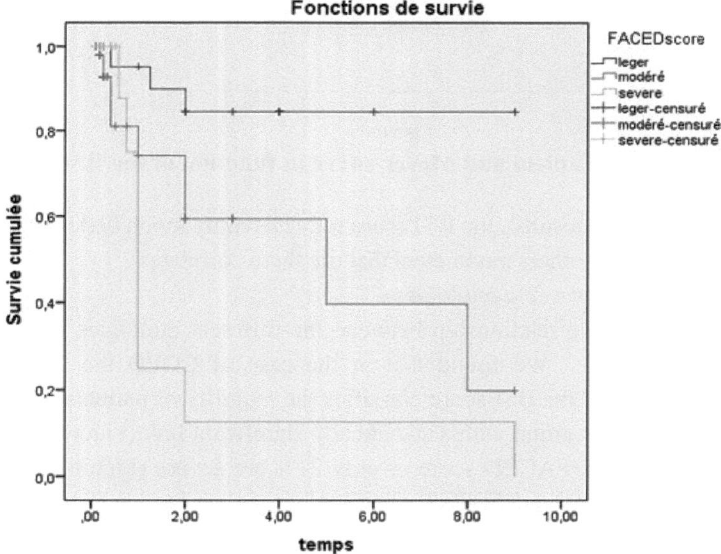

Figure 21: Kaplein and Meyer curve in function of FACED score

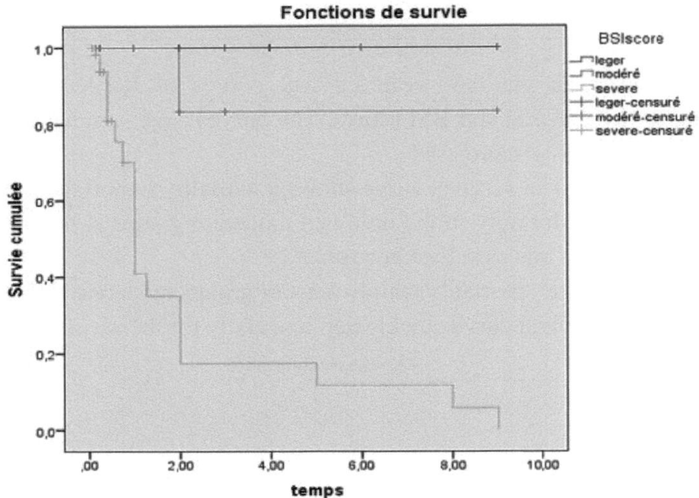

Figure 22: Kaplein and Meyer curve in function of the BSI score

According to these results , the BSI score reflects reality much better . For this , we will to research others parameters that are there correlates .

1.4.2.8 Severity scores and etiologies

We have studies the relationship between the different etiologies of DDB and the severity scores . We found that in the case of COPD the 2 scores are divergent . In fact , the BSI score classifies the majority of patients with COPD (81%) to the severe group with a statistically significant link (Figure 23). This is not the case for the FACED score or only 21% are severe (Figure 24). For the rest of the etiologies, no difference was found .

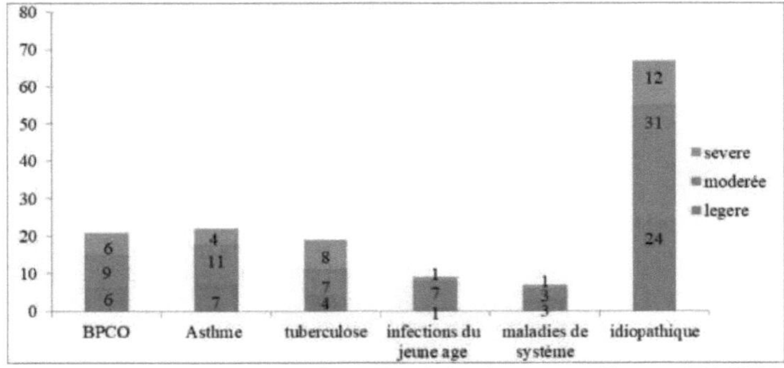

Figure 23: Distribution of DDB etiologies according to FACED

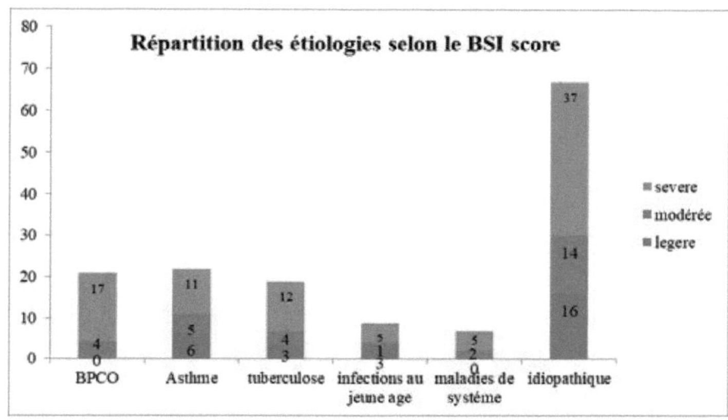

Figure 24: Distribution of etiologies according to the BSI score

Severity and impairment scores radiological :

We searched a possible relationship between the type of bronchiectasis , the number of affected lobes , lymphadenopathy hilar and mediastinal and emphysema with FACED and BSI scores. Our results have summer in favor of a statistically significant relationship between an association of 2 or more types of DDB with the 2 scores. But this relationship has summer different depending on the score used .

In fact , if we used the FACED we would have 30 patients with severity classes moderate while the BSI classifies more patients (37 cases) among the severe (Figures 25 and 26). The BSI score reflects Thus better severity radiological .

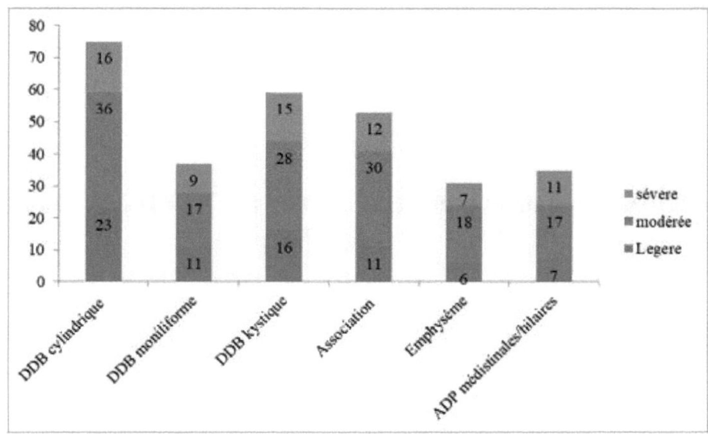

Figure 25: Distribution of lesions radiological according to the FACED score

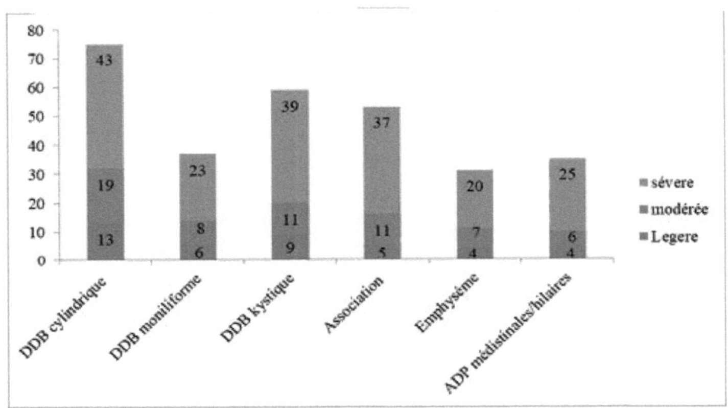

Figure 26: Distribution of lesions radiological according to the BSI score

Severity scores and FEV1

statistical link has was significant between the FEV1 value and the two severity scores (p<0.001).

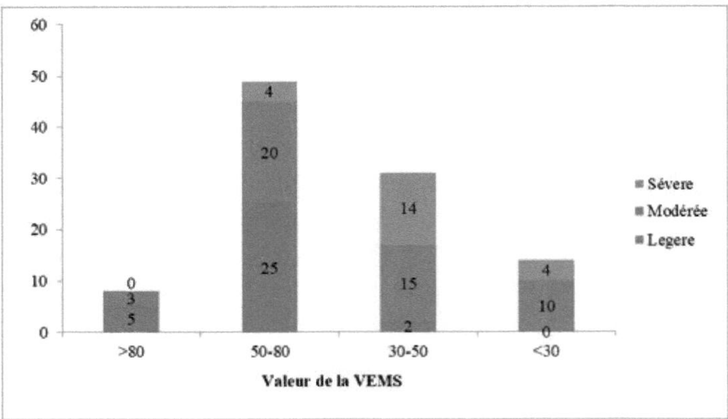

Figure 27: Distribution of patients according to FACED score and FEV1

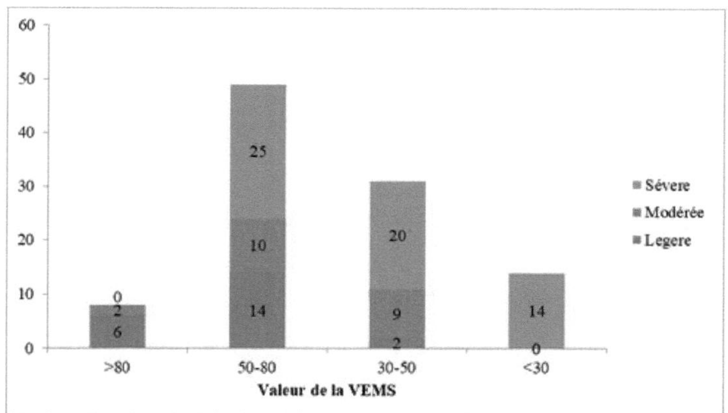

Figure 28: Distribution of patients according to BSI score and FEV1

1.4.2.11 Severity scores and Quality of life

The quality of life has summer estimated based on the SGRQ . We have calculates the 3 components of the score: symptoms , activity and impact in order to to obtain the SGRQ total. For this , we have excluded from our population the sick deaths in whom the questionnaire was not do . Thus , we obtain 82 patients .

Indeed , the median of the SGRQ total varies in function of the severity score used . Looking at the BSI score, the median of the highest SGRQ total was equal to 67 and corresponded to the severe group . Others groups moderate and light have had a total SGRQ equal to 50 and 47 respectively . For the FACED score, the median of the SGRQ was summer almost the same in the group moderate than severe with values respectively 65 and 64 and less of the order of 44 in the light group . (Figures 29 and 30).

We did not find a significant statistical link between the SGRQ and the severity scores , the p values have summer equal to 0.7 and 0.44 respectively for the BSI and the FACED scores (Fisher's exact test). Likewise, no statistical relationship n / A summer found between the 3 parts of the SGRQ (symptom , activity and impact) with the BSI and FACED scores (Table XVII).

On the other hand , there exists a significant statistical relationship between the SGRQ and the HAD scale , the number exacerbations and hospitalizations (Table XVIII).

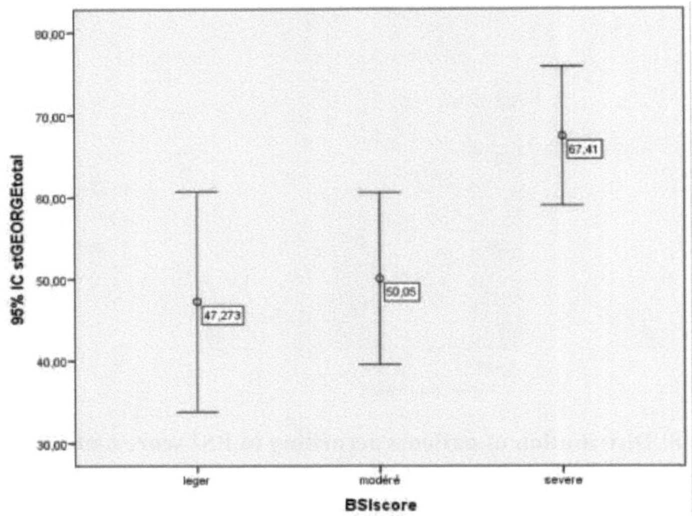

Figure 29: The total SGRQ in each severity group according to the BSI score

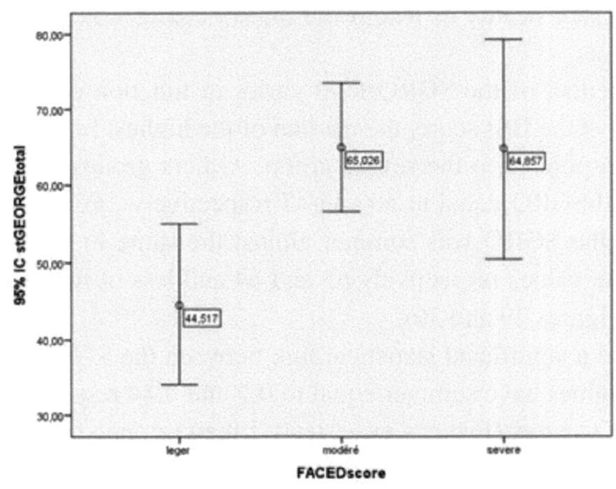

Figure 30: The total SGRQ in each severity group according to the FACED score

Table XVII: Distribution of patients according to the SGRQ and severity scores

SGRQ	Severity Score	SGRQ symptoms	SGRQ total	SGRQ impact	activity

FACED	Light 42484144	
	Modere	65646565
	Severe	65636364
BSI	Light 46514547	
	Modere	52474650
	Severe	65686867

Table XVIII: Estimated quality of life according to the SGRQ in function of severity scores

	Scale HAD	Number of exacerbations / year	Number	OLD/VNI of hospitalization / 2 years
Total SGRQ	<0.001		<0.0010,0060,001	

Severity and status scores psychological :

In order to assess the status psychological of our sick , we are based on the HAD Scale which allows devalue anxiety and depression. A total score (anxiety + depression) greater than 15 or a component (anxiety or depression) greater than 11 means the presence of an anxiety disorder Or depression in the patient . We have collects 45 patients having an anxiety- depressive disorder among 81 patients or 55.6%.

The distribution of these sick has summer different according to the severity score used . Indeed , if we used the FACED score we would have 27 patients (60 %) in the class moderate . On the other hand , in using the BSI score, we would have 27 patients classified in the severe group . (Table XIX)

statistical relationship has was significant between the HAD Scale and the 2 severity scores , the " p value " was of the order of 0.004 and 0.039 respectively for the FACED and BSI score.

Table XIX: Estimation of status psychological by the HAD scale according to severity scores

Severity Score		Positive HAD scale
FACED	Light	9
	moderately	27
	severity	9
BSI	Light	8
	moderately	10
	severity	27

1.4.3 Multivariate study of mortality

logistical regression binary has summer used to look for risk factors independent of mortality in our population. We have finds 8 factors : the number of comorbidities , GERD, asthma associates , HTA, the level socioeconomic medium to high , the number hospitalizations /2 years, isolation of Branhamella catarrhalis, non- use of Bromhexine.

Table XX: Mortality risk factors after multivariate study

Variables	HAS	RR (95% CI)	Value P
Sex	-1.61	0.58	0.45
Age	-0.054	0.28	0.59
Level socioeconomic pupil	3.58	36.37	0.006
Level socioeconomic AVERAGE	2.77	13.33	0.038
BMI	-0.67	0.000	0.62
HT	2.6	3.6	0.3
Diabetes	-0.2	0.00	0.996
COPD	-1.58	0.13	0.71
Asthma	-4.011	3,032	0.082
Heart disease ischemic	-1.05	0.01	0.998
RGO	-4.71	0.012	0.005
Name of comorbidities	1.14	6.13	0.001
CCI	0.44	0.29	0.59
Abondance de I'hemoptysie	12-13	1.14	0.77
I'hemoptysie recurrence	0.14	1.5	0.88
Branhamella Catarrhalis	1.44	1.39	0.24
Hospitalizations /2 years	-1.72	1.33	0.25
Interval hospitalizations	4.75	3.15	0.043
Exacerbations/1 year	-0.46	0.13	0.71
Bromhexine (not used)	1.06	2.89	0.27

4 Discussion

1. Epidemiology

1.1 Impact

Depending on the country

DDB is a problem health major public in Tunisia and everywhere in the world responsible of a significant health expenditure . Indeed , this permanent pathology long time under diagnosis until the advent of the chest scanner multibarettes which played a major role in his diagnosis.

In Europe, the number hospitalization for DDB is in clear rise with an average of 2.9% per year in Germany between 2005 and 2011 (18). In Spain it is estimates that the prevalence of DDB varies between 42 and 566/100,000 inhabitants.(14)

In the United Kingdom , the prevalence of BDD among women has increased increases from 350.5 per 100,000 inhabitants in 2004 to 566.1 per 100,000 inhabitants in 2013 and among men from 301.2 per 100,000 inhabitants in 2004 to 485.5 per 100,000 inhabitants in 2013 (2).

In the United States , Seitz et al (2012) reports an increase in annual prevalence arriving at 8.7% (19).

South Korea (20), the incidence of DDB is estimated to reach 464/100,000 inhabitants. From this done , we consider that DDB is not rare especially since the cost of healthcare expenditure per year reaches 218 EUR in these sick .

In Tunisia , despite recent studies carried out on this pathology , none of among She n / A estimates the true prevalence of DDB. Which is known It is what it is a common cause hospitalization in pulmonology .

Our study focused on 110 cases of diffuse DDB followed in the pulmonology department of the Hedi Chaker hospital in Sfax.

According to gender

The attack on sex male has was predominated in our study contrary to what the literature reports . In Europe, a meta analysis (10) concerning 7 cohorts Europeans (Scotland, Ireland , Italy, Belgium, Greece, England , Serbia) showed the predominance of sex female in all cohorts . Likewise, in the United States (USA) the register American research on bronchial dilation (21) counted 1826 cases of BDD collected between 2008 and 2014, 76% of which were sex. feminine . A selection bias can explain this difference since we We are particularly interested in diffuse DDBs which could influence the results .

Table XXI: Distribution by sex in the series

	Period study	Man(%)	Female(%)
Our study	2009-2019	58	42
Scotland	2011-2015	39.3	60.7
Ireland	2008-2015	32.9	67.1

Italy	2011-2015	41.2	58.8
Belgium	2006-2012	49	51
Greece	2010-2015	36	64
Anglettaire	2009-2013	40.5	59.5
Serbia	2010-2015	29.2	70.8
USA	2008-2014	24	76

<u>According to age</u>

The system immune East less effective in young children and elderly subjects , which leads to an increased incidence of infection in these two groups (22). The DDB was most often described as beginning in childhood, particularly in the first five years of life with a tendency to improve significantly in late adolescence and then a worsening of symptoms at the age of 50 to 60 years (23,24). From our days , we describe this pathology more significant in older subjects (22).

In Europe, the age average of patients with BDD ranges between 59 and 66 years according to the meta analysis which concerned 7 cohorts European (10).

In the United States , the register American research on bronchial dilation has highlighted a average age 64±14 years. The age group predominant was between 50 and 79 years old (21).

In our study, the age AVERAGE has was 60 years old with extremes ranging from 16 to 90 years and a peak frequency in the age group over 70 years old.

Table XXII: Age average of patients according to series

Series	**Period study**	**Middle age**
Our study	2009-2019	60
Scotland	2011-2015	65.3
Ireland	2008-2015	60.5
Italy	2011-2015	65.1
Belgium	2006-2012	66.4
Greece	2010-2015	59.3
England	2009-2013	59.1
Serbia	2010-2015	62
USA	2008-2014	64

1.2 Clinical study

1.2.1 Habits (smoking)

Active and passive exposure to tobacco smoke is well known as important risk factor for respiratory diseases chronicles .

In Europe a meta analysis interested 7 cohorts European prospective: Monza, Italy; Dundee and New Castle, United Kingdom ; Leuven, Belgium; Barcelona ,

Spain ; Athens, Greece; Galway, Ireland . She studied 1258 cases of DDB , 36% of which had a history of smoking (25).
In Turkey , a prospective study was carried out conducted by Onen et al regarding 98 cases of DDB (12). It showed that 24.5% of patients were tobacco with a average of 8.69±18.11 PA.
In the United States , the percentage of smoking has summer estimated at 40% (21).
Concerning our study, smoking is more common than in the literature arriving at 45% with a average of 26 AP. This can be explained by the increasingly high smoking rate . The withdrawal only interested 24 people .

1.2.2 Personal history

In the United Kingdom , Jennifer et al have studied 18,793 cases of DDB between 2004 and 2013. It showed that 63.4% of patients having one DDB had at least a disease concomitant . Among which asthma was the most common pathology (42.5%) followed by COPD (36.1%) (2).
In Turkey , patients had at least a comorbidity in 53% of cases of which a disease cardiovascular (19.4%), hypertension (21.4%) and diabetes (5.1%).
In Europe, Sara et al find that COPD associated with DDB concerns 15% of cases or that asthma has summer less common (3, 25).
In our study, personal medical history is common , reaching 84% of cases . GERD has summer the most common antecedent (29%). Other antecedents have summer reports notably hypertension (27%), asthma (20%), COPD (19%), diabetes (17%) and finally cardiovascular ATCD (coronary artery disease and arrhythmia or conduction) in 15% of cases .
In fact , gastroesophageal reflux disease (GERD) is not not uncommon during respiratory pathologies chronicles . In Australia , the prevalence of both symptomatic and symptomatic GERD or not has summer estimated by Lee et al between 26 to 75% with a significant frequency of micro aspiration of the liquid gastric in the tracheal tree bronchial (26).
Based on the different comorbidities , the Charlson score was established . Thirteen patients have had a negative CCI , the majority of patients have had a score between 1 and 4 (66%).

1.2.3 Reason for consultation

In the United States , the register American research on DDB (21) described the main symptoms reported by patients : cough (73%) which is productive in 53% of cases , dyspnea (64%), fatigue (50%).
In Europe, a meta- analysis showed that 75% of patients had a cough chronic , 62% a bronchorrhea morning , 15% a hemoptysis (25).
These results are different from ours due to the variability of symptoms during

DDB . Indeed , in our population , dyspnea of effort was predominant (99%). Cough productive chronic is Also common (82%), as is bronchorrhea morning (46%), pain thoracic infections (31%), lower respiratory infections (26%), and finally hemoptysis (25%). This difference can be explained by change epidemiological and etiological according to the origin geography of patients in the world (27).

1.3 Paraclinical study

1.3.1 Imaging thoracic : Contribution of thoracic CT multibarettes

chest scanner multibarettes represented currently the GOLD standard in the diagnosis of BDD. He plays also an important role in determining the severity of the disease since he constitutes an element of the FACED and BSI score.

1.3.1.1 Number of affected lobes

In our study, we were particularly interested in DDBs distributed with a primary aim epidemiological since these are majority in the
world and in our country. Indeed , in a multicenter study , Lynch et al have found that the localized DDB represents only 5% of the population (28). The results were no different in the United States where only 11% of patients had a localized DDB (21). Likewise, a Spanish meta- analysis (8) showed a average of affected lobes around 2.52 ±1.2.

Second , our interest in DDB, particularly diffuse, is justified since this one seems be more severe according to the literature (23).

1.3.1.2 DDB types

The identification of the three types of DDB (cylindrical , moniliform , cystic) involves nonetheless little interest clinical and does not guide the assessment etiological . On the other hand , bronchiectasis cystic are associated with a worse prognosis in terms of decline functional , sputum purulence and growth of Pseudomonas Aeruginosa (28).

In our study, the cylindrical DDBs are predominant (75%), followed by forms cystic (56%). Emphysema can be found during the DDB, Loubeyre et al (29) have demonstrated in a retrospective study carried out in France that 45% of patients had emphysema associated with DDB lesions while highlighting the relationship between emphysema and extension radiological and severity of DDB. In our study, emphysema is common reaching 30.4% of patients this can be due on the one hand to the extension radiological since we We are interested in diffuse BDD and on the other hand in the non-negligible prevalence of associated COPD (15%).

1.3.2 Cytobacteriological examination of sputum (ECBC)

The infection respiratory constitutes an evolutionary turning point in the future of the DDB from which the interest to identify the microorganisms on the patient 's sputum and this either during the exacerbations that the stable state to search a probable colonization (30).

Pseudomonas Aeruginosa and Haemophilus influenzae (HI) are the two most common bacteria isolated at scale worldwide although the proportions vary depending on the countries and populations (27). A meta analysis made by Finchk et al (31) in 2015 about 3683 patients with BDD showed that 21.4% of patients had a colonization by pyocyanin and that in these patients , mortality , frequency of hospitalizations as well as exacerbations were multiplied by three compared to non- colonized subjects . More recently in 2019, a prospective study was carried out carried out by Amorim et al (30), it showed that colonization by HI and Pseudomonas Aeruginosa was frequent in Portugal reaching respectively 32.3% and 30.1%.

Our results are different from those in the literature . Indeed , colonization by Pseudomonas Aeruginosa was identified in 4 patients only or 3.6%. On the other hand , a history of superinfection by the same germ without being able to complete the definition of colonization represents 17.3% of our population. These results can be explain since in the majority of cases and particularly in a stable state , the request for an ECBC is not common practice.

Functional exploration respiratory

She must be carried out in a stable state , outside of the surges infectious . Patients with bronchiectasis do not present a profile particular functional . The anomalies observed reflect the extension of the lesions, their severity and possible respiratory illnesses associated .

According to the recommendations Spanish studies of 2018 (14), an obstructive syndrome is observed in most patients, particularly in subjects tobacco and/ or suffering from COPD. The association has a restrictive syndrome East frequent , generally due to the presence of territories atelectasis or not ventilated due to obstructive secretions , this can be seen during tuberculosis pulmonary and in the forms fibrosing destructive .

Measuring FEV1 is essential to calculate severity scores . A meta analysis (25) showed a median FEV1 is 73%. A prospective study in Brazil (32) showed a value mean FEV1 was 48±14.8%.

In Tunisia , we do not have other studies evaluating the profile functional of patients suffering from BDD. Our results are not different from those in the literature since the ventilatory disorder obstructive is predominant in 44.5% of cases , the restrictive disorder in this way least 27.3%. The value average FEV1 in our population is 52%.

2. La mortality

Until Currently , we do not have enough studies on mortality during of the

DDB. This pathology which has summer considered without seriousness previously is no longer so today , since recent studies showed its impact on the survival of patients as well as on their quality of life.
Loebinger et al (5) have could follow patients with DDB on a period of 14 years in a study validating the SGRQ in the DDB. The authors have could describe in a manner detailed the impact of DDB on mortality : 29.7% of patients are deaths during follow - up , this value was double that expected according to life expectancy in individuals in United Kingdom . The cause of death was respiratory in 70.4% of cases .
Other studies have shown a mortality important linked to the DDB in particular in Turkey (16.3%) with a survival average estimated at 44.06±1.6 months (12). In Belgium (33), a study showed a prevalence of DDB of 539 cases among 20,998 patients consulting for disease respiratory or 2.6%. Mortality has summer important reaching 10.6%.
On the other hand , in Germany , mortality remains stable between 2005 and 2011, estimated at 0.003/100,000 inhabitants which is a value bass (18).
South Korea , it is estimated a mortality of 2.9 % intrahospital among patients having DDB and 1.4% die from DDB specifically (20).
In Tunisia , we did not find studies that allow to assess mortality linked to the DDB. Our results are similar to those in the literature , mortality high of around 19.1%. Risk factors for mortality have summer studied and will be details subsequently .

Table XXIII : Mortality according to the series

Series	Kingdom United	Türkiye	Belgium	South Korea	Our study
Period study	1994	2000-2005	2006-2009	2012-2017	2018-2019
Number of cases	111	98	539	1,400,000	110
Mortality (%)	29.7	16.3	10.6	2.9	19.1

3. The elements of prognosis

Several factors can influence the severity of DDB. We can cite the factors epidemiological as age , sex , comorbidities , factors clinics , function pulmonary , radiological abnormalities , genetics , microbiology and inflammation systemic . All these factors have been well studied in a literature review (34) and have was summarized in Table XXIV.

Table XXIV : factors influencing the prognosis of DDB in the literature

Settings clinics	Elements of a good prognosis or light DDB	Elements of bad prognosis or severe DDB
Bacteriology	No germs	**Pseudomonas Aeruginosa**

	Absence of colonization by HI	Staphylococci Aureus Methy R Enterobacteria Gram Negative Bacterial load high
Radiology	< 3 lobes Cylindrical DDBs	**> 3 lobes** **Cystic DDBs** **Wall thickening bronchial** **Infusion in mosaic** **Emphysema** Mucus plugs
Function Respiratory	Normal EFR	**Ventilatory disorder obstructive** Ventilatory disorder restrictive VR/ High CPT low DLCO
Dyspnea of effort	No Dvspnee of effort	**Dyspnea stadium 4/5 CRM**
Symptoms	Sputum volume < 5 ml/day Mucous sputum Or mucus purulent Cough occasional Or during exacerbations	Sputum volume >25 ml/day **Stable purulent sputum** Cough persistent
Etiology	No comorbidities	**Associated COPD** Associate PR
Exacerbations	<3/year	>3/year **Severe exacerbations requiring a hospitalization**

3.1 Epidemiological elements

3.1.1 Age and sex

Loebinger et al (5) have studies mortality risk factors linked to the DDB on a period of 13 years. They have found that 29.7% of patients die while normally the percentage death estimate by the national statistics office is 14.7% in men and 8.9% in women of the same age. In patients deaths by DDB, the average age is 60 years old. A multivariate study concluded that age and sex male are risk factors independent of mortality .

In Germany , Felix et al (18) have studies the frequency of hospitalization linked to DDB. According to the authors, the highest value was 39.4 hospitalizations /100,000 inhabitants and this among men aged between 75 and 84. German statistics have also shows that there were 164 deaths reported due to BDD including 93 men and 71 women . Among the sick died , 131 subjects (80%) were aged >65 and 80 (49%) were aged >70 years.

Likewise in Turkey , Onen et al (12) showed that the age average of patients died was significantly higher than survivors : 72 versus 59.7 years . The results of the multivariate study have confirms that the age is a risk factor independent of mortality , this it's not the case regarding sex .

Our study is consistent with the literature , the age AVERAGE has summer statistically higher in patients died . Mortality increases with age but after multivariate study age is not a risk factor independent of mortality . The distribution of deaths according to sex showed a predominance of sex masculine in a non-significant way . The study multivariate concludes that sex is not a risk factor for mortality .

3.1.2 Comorbidities

As with COPD, DDB can be associated with a Or several comorbidities which condition the prognosis of the disease . It is for this reason that teams were interested in to study That relation. Indeed , Melissa et al (35) highlighted that the number and nature of comorbidities are risk factors for mortality in patients followed for DDB. Mortality increases by 17% each time addition of a comorbidity . The number of comorbidities identifies reached 81 of which 13 have summer considered potentially associated with a increased mortality , which have summer included subsequently in a BACI score (Bronchiectasis **A etiology C** omorbidity **Index**). Among these comorbidities , we can cite those estimated significantly associated with mortality such as COPD, metastatic cancer , connective tissue disease , asthma , inflammatory diseases chronic digestive tract. The men had significantly more comorbidities compared to women with median of 4 comorbidities .

COPD

The association between COPD and DDB is become a subject of debate currently and has summer identifies as a particular phenotype associated with a susceptibility to tract colonization respiratory , has a increase in symptoms respiratory tract with impaired quality of life and frequent exacerbations (36, 37).

Comorbidities cardiovascular

Concerning our population, comorbidities are instead cardiovascular notably diabetes , hypertension , heart disease ischemic . The coexistence of cardiac pathologies increases the difficulty of grip caring for the sick notably in period of exacerbations or the 2 pathologies can be involved . On the other hand, the association of several risk factors cardiovascular including diabetes increases the risk of cardiac decompensation .

-esophageal reflux

Gastroesophageal reflux is common in our population, it represents a risk factor for mortality which is independent according to the study multivariate . These results are consistent with the literature as in testifies Mandal et al (38), GERD is a factor independent of risk exacerbation and severity of DDB. In addition, a study carried out by McDonnell et al (39) showed that GERD exists in 26-75%

of cases in patients having a DDB. These sick have a more severe DDB. On the other hand , the effect of GERD treatment on the prognosis of DDB is not not yet established .

Charlson's score is considered among the best known and most used comorbidity scores in chronic pathologies , cited in more than 9,500 publications. Seitz et al (19) clearly showed according to their prospective study, in 2010 that the Charlson score is a predictor of the cost student linked to care in the United States . The authors specified that the ICC can be useful for identifying patients who will to have a healthcare expenditure high .

Our results are consistent with those in the literature with a statistically significant relationship between mortality and CCI during the study bivariate (p=0.004) but this connection is not significant in the study multivariate (p=0.54).

On the other hand, go assess the number of comorbidities East interesting . In our study we found a significant statistical link with mortality After the study multivariate (p= 0.001). Thus the number of comorbidities is a risk factor independent of mortality whatever the comorbidity .

3.2 Clinical elements

The DDB is a pathology disabling , the signs clinics respiratory are common and may resist treatment pharmacological . Several studies have been interested in determining the symptoms respiratory associated with increased severity of the disease while emphasizing the importance to evaluate the quality of life among these sick . Among the signs clinical , dyspnea effort and sputum volume have summer described in several publications.

As in testifies Martinez-Garda et al (6) in a prospective study of 86 patients that dyspnea effort and sputum volume (in milliliters) are significantly correlated with the SGRQ (multivariate study).

On the other hand, MP Murray et al (40) have studies the relationship between the color of sputum and the severity of the disease . According to the authors, a colonization bacteria affects 5% of sputum mucous ; 43.5% of sputum mucopurulent and 86.4% of sputum purulent in a stable state . They have could demonstrate After analysis multivariate as sputum purulent are linked to several factors independent including colonization bacterial , cystic BDD , FEV <80% and age of onset of disease before age 45.

Our study did not demonstrate a relationship between the symptoms clinical and mortality even after multivariate study .

3.3 Radiological elements

There is no radiological score specific for non- cystic fibrosis DDB . It exists nevertheless many other scores for cystic fibrosis and which have summer a long time used for non- cystic fibrosis DDB . Among these scores the Reiff modifies (41) allows to study the severity of the dilation (1= cylindrical ; 2= moniliform ; 3= cystic) as well as the number of lobes affected. This score is simple and correlates with the severity of the disease especially colonization by Pseudomonas Aeruginosa.

On the other hand , its main limitation remains the simplicity of this score as in testify Loubeyre et al (29) that the prognosis of the disease depends on other factors radiological : wall thickness bronchial , mucous plugs , infusion mosaic and emphysema pulmonary .

Other scores have summer use like the Bhalla score (42) which takes taking into consideration the presence of bubbles , atelectasis etc. This score has summer subsequently validated for non - cystic fibrosis DDB and was well correlated with disease prognosis . The Brody and Robinson scores did not yet been valid during non- cystic fibrosis DDB .

In our study we did not use these radiological scores since we We are interested in the two FACED scores and BSI scores which allow to evaluate , among other things, the factors radiological notably the number of lobes for the two scores and the type of bronchiectasis (cystic) for the BSI.

Furthermore , no statistical relationship was found between the severity of the disease and the radiological elements .

3.4 Microbiological elements

Colonization by Pseudomonas Aeruginosa is associated with a more severe BDD with a greater decline in FEV1 and a higher mortality (31, 43). Several studies emphasize the benefit of performing ECBC in a stable state to look for pyocyanin with the aim of eradicating it (44). The impact on the quality of life for this germ has summer Also demonstrated by Wilson et al (45).

In our work, contrary to the literature , no correlation was found summer found between mortality and colonization by pyocyanic . The number reduces sickness colonized in our population can influence our results .

On the other hand, although isolated in 5 patients only , superinfection with Moraxella catarrhalis is a risk factor independent of mortality after multivariate study .

3.5 The etiologies

The DDB is a pathology heterogeneous , however her occurrence supposes the conjunction of factors environmental, especially infectious , and a predisposing terrain . Variability between different continents summer widely incriminated and this was illustrated in figure (27).

In the literature , based on a meta analysis Chinese made by YOUNG-HUA et al (46) and on a Spanish multicenter study (47) we have believes that the origin infectious of which tuberculosis and infections at young age are the most incriminated (30%) then that DDB associated with respiratory diseases chronicles East found from 6.3% to 13.7%. Tuberculosis pulmonary represents 18.6% of etiologies in Spain .

By focusing on respiratory diseases chronic , the association of COPD and DDB is not rare, it represents 3.9 to 7.8%. In addition, this association has summer considered as a separate phenotype, associated with frequent exacerbations , with a clinical representation quite rich and has a prognosis bad . Among the sick having severe COPD , associated DDB East found in 30 to 50% of cases and the prevalence of BDD increases with the severity of COPD. Concerning asthma , a less association frequents 1.4 to 5.4%. Among asthmatics severe or uncontrolled , it is estimated that 20 to 30% have an associated DDB . The causal relationship is unknown until now. At these patients we must rule out the diagnosis of ABPA.

Other etiologies should be cited such as immune deficiency which represents 5 - to 9.4% and thus less systemic diseases (1.4-3.8 %) or polyarthritis rheumatoid has summer a long time estimated responsible for a bad prognosis justifying close monitoring during visits medical according to the recommendations of BTS (48).

The DDB is idiopathic when all investigation etiological comes back negative, it represents 24.2-44.8% of cases .

In Tunisia , there is no study on the relationship between mortality and the etiologies of DDB. Our results are not as different from the literature . Indeed , idiopathic DDB represented a good part in 65% of cases . The etiologies that we found have summer characterized by their variability but none n / A summer correlated with mortality . On the other hand , COPD is associated with a more severe DDB according to the BSI score and this it's not the case if we used the FACED score.

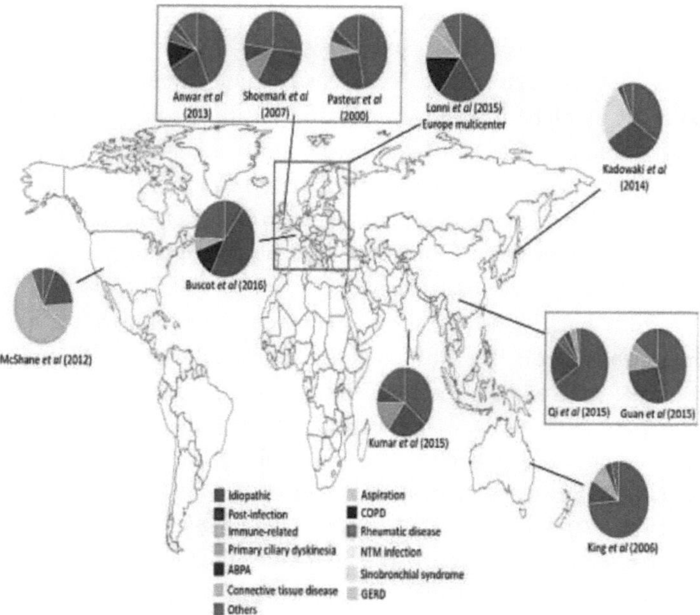

Chandrasekaran R et al Geographic variation in the aetiology , epidemiology and microbiology of bronchiectasis. BMC Pulm Med. Dec 2018

Figure 31: Etiologies of DDB in the world according to geographic and ethnic origin

4. Severity scores : ultimately BSI or FACED score?

Until today two severity scores have summer valid in non- cystic fibrosis DDB : FACED and BSI. Both have advantages and disadvantages . The FACED score is easier to calculate and interpret since it contains 5 dichotomous variables . On the other hand , the BSI score is relatively complex putting in sets of 9 non-dichotomous variables and with precise values for each .

Both classify the sick in 3 categories according to the degree of severity of the disease with a good prediction of mortality but in a way different . Indeed , FACED has was developed to predict mortality at 5 years while the BSI was developed in addition to estimating mortality , to predict exacerbations and in particular those requiring a hospitalization and estimate quality of life .

Several studies have summer made with the aim of comparing the two scores on different populations . No study has summer done in Tunisia despite the increase in the prevalence of the disease and health expenditure , especially during hospitalizations .

Mac Donnell et al (10) were interested in a meta analysis doing include 7 cohorts European in 2016, comparing the 2 scores on 1612 patients . According

to the authors, the 2s scores make it possible to predict mortality but the BSI is clearly superior in predicting exacerbations, quality of life, symptoms respiratory , physical exercise and decline in function respiratory .
A second study summer Also done in 2016 by Ellis et al (11) over 19 years of monitoring and allowed to study the prediction of long- term mortality . At 5 years old the two scores allow a good prediction of mortality . At 15 years old , the two scores allow also predict mortality but with a better predictive value for the FACED score compared to the BSI. The weak point of this study was the weak number of the sample (91 patients).
In 2017, a study by JC Costa et al (49) allowed us to compare the two scores. According to the authors, the BSI tends to classify patients mainly in the severe group and they have explain these results by the higher number of variables of the BSI compared to the FACED. The weak points of this study are : the number limit of the sample (40 patients) and that it there were no deaths during the study preventing thus the authors studied mortality .
Edmundo et al (50) have led a study in 2017 on a larger sample (198 patients) but with a methodology different . In fact , they have divides the population into 2 categories: Frequent exacerbator (>2 exacerbations/year) and mild exacerbator (< exacerbations/year). They then studied the FACED and BSI scores in each category . The ill Frequent exacerbators have risk factors like a more advanced age , a colonization by Pseudomonas Aeruginosa, low FEV1 and Tiffneau ratio values and an association with COPD. On the other hand, if we look at the BSI and FACED scores, age , Pseudomonas Aeruginosa are the 2 elements involved in the frequency of exacerbations, and we add for the BSI the notion of a hospitalization and exacerbation anterior .

4.1 Comparison according to mortality prediction

According to our results , the BSI score is more sensitive in predicting mortality than the FACED score. AUC values are different with a significant AUC for the BSI score (0.77) but not significant for the FACED (0.67).
If we are going to base ourselves on the BSI score, the Kaplein and Meyer survival curves are in favor of a survival at 10 years which is unfavorable especially for the severe group . The survival is on the other hand better for the group weak to moderate . In this case , the BSI is a good tool allowing us to discern between patients in front require a socket support enough thrust (severe group) and those including monitoring can be done with a family doctor (mild group). On the other hand, in looking at the Kaplein and Meyer curve for the FACED score, we find that mortality increases especially in both groups moderate and severe. This discrepancy between the BSI and the FACED score is due to the difference in their variables and in the allocation of points for each

variable. Indeed , in analyzing mortality risk factors according to our study, we find that some factors are included in the BSI score and not in the FACED such as the BMI which can explain this discrepancy in results for our population. On the other hand, when we interested in parameters composing the two scores, the values attributed to the same variable differ depending on the score used . We We are interested in variables that have constitutes a risk factor independent of mortality as we quote:

* **For Page** : the BSI score holds in has 4 age groups with values arriving at 6 points over 80 years old , 4 points over 70 years old and 2 points from 50 years old. These values important influence the total score and age alone, rated at 6 points, already classifies the DDB as moderate . As for the FACED score, age over 70 years old takes 2 points and the age rated at 2 points classifies the DDB as mild . A sick meme will be classified Thus differently depending on whether we apply the BSI or the FACED.

* **For dyspnea of effort** : the classification was base mainly on the MRC for the BSI and mMRC for the FACED. Values attributed arrive has 3 points for stage 5 MRC for the BSI but for the FACED it East lesser arriving at 1 point for stage 3 and 4 mMRC .

* **For FEV1** : the FACED score assigns for all value <50% 2 points while the BSI awards 3 points for FEV <30% and 1 point for an FEV between 50 and 80%. FEV1 which is a factor in mortality independent East thus underestimated by the FACED score unlike the BSI.

4.2 Comparison according to the prediction of hospitalizations and exacerbations

The two scores are risk predictions hospitalization with an AUC >0.7 for each. Furthermore , the BSI score is more sensitive in predicting hospitalizations than the FACED score since the AUC corresponding was 0.95 versus 0.69 for the FACED score (p<0.0001). In the litterature an AUC >0.8 is considered excellent which constitutes a strong point for the BSI. These results can be explained by the fact that the BSI score includes Already among its variables a hospitalization within 2 years previous ones . On the other hand, the BSI attributes 5 points to this variable, this value allow straight away to classify the DDB as moderate . We consider that this value East overrated if we are faced with a excessive hospitalization in some case individuals (best access to care) while the DDB is Normally light if we did not take this into account postman .

The two scores do not allow a good prediction of exacerbations. Although the BSI holds in account This factor and assigns 2 points beyond 3 exacerbations. Only 29% of patients are considered by the BSI to have had exacerbations exceeding 3/year. We consider than a good interrogation is necessary to detect the number exact exacerbations since the patient can miss an exacerbation and this have the BSI score results modified . A score has summer established by Martinez Garcia et al (51) called EXA-FACED to compensate for FACED taking into account the exacerbations factor . This is a score that has shown good predictive value for exacerbations and mortality .

4.3 Comparison according to quality of life

The DDB is a disease heterogeneous and quite complex . Therefore the severity of this pathology necessarily involves assessing the quality of life . The SGRQ is a valid and long-lasting questionnaire used during respiratory pathologies chronicles like COPD but also the DDB.

A metaanalysis made by Spinou et al (52) in 2016 about 43 studies (3727 patients having a DDB). The authors were interested in the questionnaires used in estimating the quality of life among these sick . They have concluded that the SGRQ is the most used (63%) and the most associated with dyspnea of effort . Nevertheless , it is a score considered long and difficult for the patient to complete . A more recent study in 2018 made by Dudgeon et al (53) on a sample reduced (8 patients) and which made it possible to conclude that the SGRQ presents 3 negative points according to the participants: some questions are difficult , the control of the questionnaire after 3 months and the questions using true /false which are not precise.

According to a study done in 2013 by Charrier et al (54), after 6 months of respiratory rehabilitation , they noted a significant improvement in the quality of life of patients in using the SGRQ score.

For our population, we have calculated this questionnaire among survivors , the results did not show any difference between the two scores. In fact , severe class patients have a total SGRQ of around 67 and 65 respectively for the BSI and the FACED score. No correlation has summer established between the scores and the SGRQ. The negative point of this questionnaire is the number of parts (3 parts) and high questions can be enough heavy to complete by the patient and the doctor . Other questionnaires have summer established

4.4 Status psychological

Detecting anxiety-depressive disorders could prove necessary in a process of taking overall care of a patient presenting a DDB. As in testify Bousoffara et al (55) in a Tunisian prospective study led in 2014: the prevalence of depression was 20.8 % and that of anxiety 22.7% in using the HAD scale . The authors have finds that the sick having an anxiety-depressive disorder had a dyspnea more advanced effort , low FEV1 and rapid progression towards insufficiency respiratory chronicle . Nevertheless It is a study that takes in counts patients without comorbidities associates which is not the case in our study.

On the other hand, Olveira et al (56) have studies the relationship showed that symptoms of depression and anxiety are factors independent of a bad quality of life of patients.
In our study, 45 patients have an anxiety-depressive disorder among 81 patients or 55.6%.
The distribution of these sick has summer different according to the severity score used . Indeed , if we used the FACED score we would have 27 patients (60 %) in the class moderate . On the other hand , in using the BSI score, we would have 27 patients classified in the severe group .
statistical relationship has was significant between the HAD Scale and the 2 severity scores , the " p value " was of the order of 0.004 and 0.039 respectively for the FACED and BSI score.

New severity score from DDB offers:

Based on the results of the study multivariate , several mortality risk factors have been identified in our population. Some factors are not included in the BSI and FACED scores. Thus , taking into account the BSI score which is the best score applicable for our population, we propose to take into account account these risk factors identifies: The number of comorbidities all combined , the history of hypertension asthma and GERD, the level socio-economic , a superinfection by Branhamella Catarrhalis and non- use of Bromhexine.
According to the literature , inflammation systemic has summer proposed as a potential explanation of the mechanism linking DDB as for COPD to comorbidities with part of the aging process (57). Statins and macrolides have demonstrated their effectiveness during DDB according to randomized controlled studies , due to their anti- inflammatory activity . The development of new anti- inflammatory drugs selective could be promising in the future (58). On the other hand, according to our work, Bromhexine plays a protective role since the absence of this treatment presents a risk factor independent of mortality . The treatment mucolytic is routine practice, a Cochrane literature review (59) reports that only 2 studies have been interested in mycolytic agents in DDB apart or not from exacerbations but the results remain inconclusive .
Other studies will be necessary to rate the new items of the score and validate it among the Tunisian population .

Table XXV: The variables making up the new score

Variable
Age (year)
<50
50-69
70-79
>80

Body mass index (BMI)
<18.5
>18.5
FEV(%)
>80%
50-80%
30-49%
<30%
Hospitalizations in the previous 2 years
No
Yes
Exacerbations during the year previous 0-2
>3
Dyspnea - CKD
1-3
4
5
Colonization by Pseudomonas Aeruginosa No
Yes
Colonization by another microorganism
No
Yes
Radiological extension (> 3 lobes and/ or cystic DDB)
No
Yes
Level socioeconomic
Asthma
HT
GERD
Number of comorbidities
Superinfection by Branhamella Catarrhalis
Non- use of Bromhexine

The strong points of our study are :

The first strong point of this work is to focus on the DDB which is a neglected pathology and demonstrate mortality important linked to this pathology .

On the other hand, we are focused on severity scores described in the literature (BSI and FACED) which have not been studied previously on the Tunisian population and it still enhances our work.

We can also note that the analysis of the parameters reliable and valid as the SGRQ, HAD scale and the Charlson Comorbidity index are strong points of this study.

Finally analysis The statistics in this study made it possible to objectively compare the differences between the results .

Limitations of the study :

The first weak point of the study is the sample size that is weak and the retrospective type of the study .

Concerning the sick Already deaths , an estimate of their quality of life has not been made by the SGRQ which leads to a selection bias .

It should also be noted that the examination sputum cytobacteriology is not systematic in our daily practice , especially in a stable state . This will reduce the likelihood of colonization bacterial .

5 Conclusion

bronchial dilation (DDB) is a increasingly common pathology in pulmonology . Currently, we are witnessing more severe forms associated with a increased mortality . The diagnosis of DDB is easily established using chest CT multibarette , unlike the etiological and therapeutic approach which can prove difficult mainly secondary to character heterogeneity of the disease .
That's why that it seemed to us interesting to contribute through this retrospective study of 110 cases on patients collections between 2009 and 2018 in the pulmonology unit of the Hedi Chaker hospital in Sfax to analyze the factors prognostics and to compare the two severity scores BSI and FACED in order to choose the best for our population.
Our results are the following :
The data demographic showed a sex ratio of 1.4 with a male predominance (58%). Age AVERAGE was 60 years old. Smoking was present in 46% of patients .
Personal history is variable dominated by comorbidities cardiovascular diseases , GERD, asthma and COPD. Level socioeconomic was average in almost half of the cases .
clinical picture remains dominated by dyspnea of effort then productive cough and bronchorrhea morning .
Chest CT confirms the diagnosis of DDB and studies both the type of lesions. In our population, the forms cylindrical are the most common (75%) and associations between the different types are not rare (51.9%).
A microbiological study using ECBC showed 5 patients colonized by pyocyanin . On the other hand , superinfections are not rare like pyocyanic which concerned 24 patients and the others germs are present in 22 cases .
Spirometry made it possible to measure FEV1 which was in average of 52%. We also note the frequency of the ventilatory disorder obstructive in 45% of cases .
The etiologies of DDB for our population are mainly infectious. including tuberculosis (19 %) and infections at young age (9%), systemic diseases are least (7%). In the majority of cases , the DDB remains idiopathic (65%).
Prognostically :
Mortality in our population is important reaching 20.6%. It increases with age Or She reaches 13.7% over the age of 65. It predominates in sex male (25.9%) without significant relationship. In the literature , data remain limited since he is of a pathology still under diagnosis . In the United Kingdom , mortality East high reaching 29% Other studies have shown a mortality important linked to the DDB in particular in Turkey (16.3%) and in Belgium (10.6%) , South Korea (2.9% intrahospital) .

The data from our study have concluded with risk factors independent of mortality which are numerous and can be summed up as follows:

- Level socioeconomic AVERAGE has pupil
- The number of comorbidities
- Some background: HTA , Asthma , GERD
- Superinfection by Branhamella Catarrhalis
- Failure to use Bromhexine
- Hospitalizations / previous 2 years

Regarding severity scores : BSI versus FACED

For our population, the BSI score is best making it possible to predict long - term mortality . In addition, it is more sensitive in the prediction of hospitalizations which constitutes already a risk factor independent of mortality . Likewise, the BSI score has a significant statistical relationship with the decline in FEV1. On the other hand , no score makes it possible to predict exacerbations in our series . These results are expected , since in the literature the BSI score is considered by most studies sensitive in mortality as well as in the prediction of exacerbations , hospitalizations , decline in FEV1 and impairment of quality of life.

Currently, quality of life represents an essential step in estimating the severity of BDD. The SGRQ allows us to reflect the quality of life among our patients with a significant relationship with the HAD scale , the number exacerbations and hospitalizations .

6 Bibliography

1. Fuschillo S, De Felice A, Balzano G. Mucosal inflammation in idiopathic bronchiectasis: cellular and molecular mechanisms. Eur Respir J. 1 fevr 2008;31(2):396- 406.

2. Quint JK, Millett ERC, Joshi M, Navaratnam V, Thomas SL, Hurst JR, et al. Changes in the incidence, prevalence and mortality of bronchiectasis in the UK from 2004 to 2013: a populationbased cohort study. Eur Respir J. janv 2016;47(1):186- 93.

3. Goeminne PC, Hernandez F, Diel R, Filonenko A, Hughes R, Juelich F, et al. The economic burden of bronchiectasis - known and unknown: a systematic review. BMC Pulm Med. dec 2019;19(1):54.

4. King PT, Holdsworth SR, Freezer NJ, Villanueva E, Holmes PW. Characterisation of the onset and presenting clinical features of adult bronchiectasis. Respir Med. dec 2006;100(12):2183- 9.

5. Loebinger MR, Wells AU, Hansell DM, Chinyanganya N, Devaraj A, Meister M, et al. Mortality in bronchiectasis: a long-term study assessing the factors influencing survival. Eur Respir J. 1 oct 2009;34(4):843- 9.

6. Martinez-Garda MA, Perpina-Tordera M, Roman-Sanchez P, Soler-Cataluna JJ. Quality-of-Life Determinants in Patients With Clinically Stable Bronchiectasis. Chest. aout 2005;128(2):739- 45.

7. Chalmers JD, Goeminne P, Aliberti S, McDonnell MJ, Lonni S, Davidson J, et al. The Bronchiectasis Severity Index. An International Derivation and Validation Study. Am J Respir Crit Care Med. mars 2014;189(5):576- 85.

8. Martinez-Garcia MA, de Gracia J, Vendrell Relat M, Giron R-M, Maiz Carro L, de la Rosa Carrillo D, et al. Multidimensional approach to non-cystic fibrosis bronchiectasis: the FACED score. Eur Respir J. 1 mai 2014;43(5):1357- 67.

9. Athanazio R, Pereira MC, Gramblicka G, Cavalcanti-Lundgren F, de Figueiredo MF, Arancibia F, et al. Latin America validation of FACED score in patients with bronchiectasis: an analysis of six cohorts. BMC Pulm Med. dec 2017;17(1):73.

10. McDonnell MJ, Aliberti S, Goeminne PC, Dimakou K, Zucchetti SC, Davidson J, et al. Multidimensional severity assessment in bronchiectasis: an analysis of seven European cohorts. Thorax. dec 2016;71(12):1110- 8.

11. Ellis HC, Cowman S, Fernandes M, Wilson R, Loebinger MR. Predicting mortality in bronchiectasis using bronchiectasis severity index and FACED scores: a 19-year cohort study. Eur Respir J. fevr 2016;47(2):482- 9.

12. Onen ZP, Eris Gulbay B, Sen E, Akkoca Yildiz O, Saryal S, Acican T, et al. Analysis of the factors related to mortality in patients with bronchiectasis. Respir Med. juill 2007;101(7):1390- 7.

13. Minov J, Karadzinska-Bislimovska J, Vasilevska K, Stoleski S, Mijakoski D. Assessment of the Non-Cystic Fibrosis Bronchiectasis Severity: The FACED Score vs the Bronchiectasis Severity Index. Open Respir Med J. 31 mars 2015;9(1):46- 51.

14. Martmez-Garda MA, Maiz L, Olveira C, Giron RM, de la Rosa D, Blanco M, et al. Spanish Guidelines on the Evaluation and Diagnosis of Bronchiectasis in Adults. Arch Bronconeumol Engl Ed. fevr 2018;54(2):79- 87.

15. Charlson ME, Pompei P, Ales KL, MacKenzie CR. A new method of classifying prognostic comorbidity in longitudinal studies: Development and validation. J Chronic Dis. janv 1987;40(5):373- 83.

16. Jones PW, Quirk FH, Baveystock CM. The St George's Respiratory Questionnaire. Respir Med. sept 1991;85:25- 31.

17. Martmez Garcia MA, Perpina Tordera M, Roman Sanchez P, Cataluna S. Internal Consistency and Validity of the Spanish Version of the St. George' Respiratory Questionnaire for Use in Patients With Clinically Stable Bronchiectasis. Arch Bronconeumol Engl Ed. mars 2005;41(3):110- 7.

18. Ringshausen FC, de Roux A, Pletz MW, Hamalainen N, Welte T, Rademacher J. Bronchiectasis-Associated Hospitalizations in Germany, 2005-2011: A Population-Based Study of Disease Burden and Trends. Fessler MB, editeur. PLoS ONE. 1 aout 2013;8(8):e71109.

19. Seitz AE, Olivier KN, Steiner CA, Montes de Oca R, Holland SM, Prevots DR. Trends and

Burden of Bronchiectasis-Associated Hospitalizations in the United States, 1993-2006. Chest. oct 2010;138(4):944- 9.

20. Choi H, Yang B, Nam H, Kyoung D-S, Sim YS, Park HY, et al. Population-based prevalence of bronchiectasis and associated comorbidities in South Korea. Eur Respir J. aout 2019;54(2):1900194.

21. Aksamit TR, O'Donnell AE, Barker A, Olivier KN, Winthrop KL, Daniels MLA, et al. Adult Patients With Bronchiectasis. Chest. mai 2017;151(5):982- 92.

22. Sadighi Akha AA. Aging and the immune system: An overview. J Immunol Methods. dec 2018;463:21- 6.

23. Field CE. Bronchiectasis. Third report on a follow-up study of medical and surgical cases from childhood. Arch Dis Child. 1 oct 1969;44(237):551- 61.

24. King P. The pathophysiology of bronchiectasis. Int J Chron Obstruct Pulmon Dis. oct 2009;411.

25. Lonni S, Chalmers JD, Goeminne PC, McDonnell MJ, Dimakou K, De Soyza A, et al. Etiology of Non-Cystic Fibrosis Bronchiectasis in Adults and Its Correlation to Disease Severity. Ann Am Thorac Soc. dec 2015;12(12):1764- 70.

26. Lee AL, Button BM, Denehy L, Wilson JW. Gastro-Oesophageal Reflux in Noncystic Fibrosis Bronchiectasis. Pulm Med. 2011;2011:1- 6.

27. Chandrasekaran R, Mac Aogain M, Chalmers JD, Elborn SJ, Chotirmall SH. Geographic variation in the aetiology, epidemiology and microbiology of bronchiectasis. BMC Pulm Med. dec 2018;18(1):83.

28. Lynch DA, Newell J, Hale V, Dyer D, Corkery K, Fox NL, et al. Correlation of CT findings with clinical evaluations in 261 patients with symptomatic bronchiectasis. Am J Roentgenol. juill 1999;173(1):53- 8.

29. Loubeyre P, Paret M, Revel D, Wiesendanger T, Brune J. Thin-Section CT Detection of Emphysema Associated With Bronchiectasis and Correlation With Pulmonary Function Tests. Chest. fevr 1996;109(2):360- 5.

30. Amorim A, Meira L, Redondo M, Ribeiro M, Castro R, Rodrigues M, et al. Chronic Bacterial Infection Prevalence, Risk Factors, and Characteristics: A Bronchiectasis Population-Based Prospective Study. J Clin Med. 6 mars 2019;8(3):315.

31. Finch S, McDonnell MJ, Abo-Leyah H, Aliberti S, Chalmers JD. A Comprehensive Analysis of the Impact of *Pseudomonas aeruginosa* Colonisation on Prognosis in Adult Bronchiectasis. Ann Am Thorac Soc. 10 sept 2015;AnnalsATS.201506-333OC.

32. Machado BC, Jacques PS, Penteado LP, Roth Dalcin P de T. Prognostic Factors in Adult Patients with Non-Cystic Fibrosis Bronchiectasis. Lung. dec 2018;196(6):691- 7.

33. Goeminne P, Scheers H, Decraene A, Seys S, Dupont L. Risk factors for morbidity and death in non-cystic fibrosis bronchiectasis: a retrospective cross-sectional analysis of CT diagnosed bronchiectatic patients. Respir Res. 2012;13(1):21.

34. Poppelwell L, Chalmers JD. Defining severity in non-cystic fibrosis bronchiectasis. Expert Rev Respir Med. avr 2014;8(2):249- 62.

35. McDonnell MJ, Aliberti S, Goeminne PC, Restrepo MI, Finch S, Pesci A, et al. Comorbidities and the risk of mortality in patients with bronchiectasis: an international multicentre cohort study. Lancet Respir Med. dec 2016;4(12):969- 79.

36. Martinez-Garcia MA, Miravitlles M. Bronchiectasis in COPD patients: more than a comorbidity? Int J Chron Obstruct Pulmon Dis. mai 2017;Volume 12:1401- 11.

37. Labaki WW, Han MK. Impact of bronchiectasis on the frequency and severity of respiratory exacerbations in COPD. Int J Chron Obstruct Pulmon Dis. juill 2018;Volume 13:2335- 8.

38. Mandal P, Morice AH, Chalmers JD, Hill AT. Symptoms of airway reflux predict exacerbations and quality of life in bronchiectasis. Respir Med. juill 2013;107(7):1008- 13.

39. McDonnell MJ, O'Toole D, Ward C, Pearson JP, Lordan JL, De Soyza A, et al. A qualitative synthesis of gastro-oesophageal reflux in bronchiectasis: Current understanding and future risk. Respir Med. aout 2018;141:132- 43.

40. Murray MP, Pentland JL, Turnbull K, MacQuarrie S, Hill AT. Sputum colour: a useful clinical tool in non-cystic fibrosis bronchiectasis. Eur Respir J. 1 aout 2009;34(2):361- 4.
41. Reiff DB, Wells AU, Carr DH, Cole PJ, Hansell DM. CT findings in bronchiectasis: limited value in distinguishing between idiopathic and specific types. Am J Roentgenol. aout 1995;165(2):261- 7.
42. Park J, Kim S, Lee YJ, Park JS, Cho Y-J, Yoon HI, et al. Factors associated with radiologic progression of non-cystic fibrosis bronchiectasis during long-term follow-up: Radiologic progression of bronchiectasis. Respirology. aout 2016;21(6):1049- 54.
43. McDonnell MJ, Jary HR, Perry A, MacFarlane JG, Hester KLM, Small T, et al. Non cystic fibrosis bronchiectasis: A longitudinal retrospective observational cohort study of Pseudomonas persistence and resistance. Respir Med. juin 2015;109(6):716- 26.
44. Tassart G, Pieters T, Gohy S. PRISE EN CHARGE DES BRONCHECTASIES DE L'ADULTE. Rev Med Liege. :9.
45. Wilson CB, Jones PW, O'Leary CJ, Hansell DM, Cole PJ, Wilson R. Effect of sputum bacteriology on the quality of life of patients with bronchiectasis. Eur Respir J. 1 aout 1997;10(8):1754- 60.
46. Gao Y, Guan W, Liu S, Wang L, Cui J, Chen R, et al. Aetiology of bronchiectasis in adults: A systematic literature review: Aetiology in bronchiectasis. Respirology. nov 2016;21(8):1376- 83.
47. Olveira C, Padilla A, Martinez-Garcia M-A, de la Rosa D, Giron R-M, Vendrell M, et al. Etiology of Bronchiectasis in a Cohort of 2047 Patients. An Analysis of the Spanish Historical Bronchiectasis Registry. Arch Bronconeumol Engl Ed. juill 2017;53(7):366- 74.
48. T Hill A, L Sullivan A, D Chalmers J, De Soyza A, Stuart Elborn J, Andres Floto R, et al. British Thoracic Society Guideline for bronchiectasis in adults. Thorax. janv 2019;74(Suppl 1):1- 69.
49. Costa JC, Machado JN, Ferreira C, Gama J, Rodrigues C. The Bronchiectasis Severity Index and FACED score for assessment of the severity of bronchiectasis. Pulmonology. mai 2018;24(3):149- 54.
50. Rosales-Mayor E, Polverino E, Raguer L, Alcaraz V, Gabarrus A, Ranzani O, et al. Comparison of two prognostic scores (BSI and FACED) in a Spanish cohort of adult patients with bronchiectasis and improvement of the FACED predictive capacity for exacerbations. Loukides S, editeur. PLOS ONE. 6 avr 2017;12(4):e0175171.
51. Martinez-Garcia MA, Athanazio RA, Giron RM, Maiz-Carro L, de la Rosa D, Olveira C, et al. Predicting high risk of exacerbations in bronchiectasis: the E-FACED score. Int J Chron Obstruct Pulmon Dis. janv 2017;Volume 12:275- 84.
52. Spinou A, Fragkos KC, Lee KK, Elston C, Siegert RJ, Loebinger MR, et al. The validity of health-related quality of life questionnaires in bronchiectasis: a systematic review and metaanalysis. Thorax. aout 2016;71(8):683- 94.
53. Dudgeon EK, Crichton M, Chalmers JD. "The missing ingredient": the patient perspective of health related quality of life in bronchiectasis: a qualitative study. BMC Pulm Med. Dec 2018;18(1):81.
54. Charrier M. Respiratory rehabilitation and quality of life in patients with bronchial dilatation . 2013;56.
55. Boussoffara L, Boudawara N, Gharsallaoui Z, Sakka M, Knani J. Troubles anxiodepressifs et dilatation des bronches. Rev Mal Respir. mars 2014;31(3):230- 6.
56. Olveira C, Olveira G, Gaspar I, Dorado A, Cruz I, Soriguer F, et al. Depression and anxiety symptoms in bronchiectasis: associations with health-related quality of life. Qual Life Res. avr 2013;22(3):597- 605.
57. Fabbri LM, Luppi F, Beghe B, Rabe KF. Complex chronic comorbidities of COPD. Eur Respir J. 1 janv 2008;31(1):204- 12.
58. Koser U, Hill A. What's new in the management of adult bronchiectasis? F1000Research. 20 avr 2017;6:527.
59. Welsh EJ, Evans DJ, Fowler SJ, Spencer S. Interventions for bronchiectasis: an overview of

Cochrane systematic reviews. Cochrane Airways Group, editeur. Cochrane Database Syst Rev [Internet]. 14 juill 2015 [cite 30 dec 2019]; Disponible sur: http://doi.wiley.com/10.1002/14651858.CD010337.pub2

7 Annexes

Annexe 1 : Fiche de recueil de donnees

Last name First name File number

Age

Sex

BMI

Urban Rural Origin

Occupation

Habits

Active / passive tobacco Number PA

Alcohol

ATCD

Obesity

Diabetes

COPD

Asthma measles

GERD

HT

Heart disease : ischemic / rhythm disturbances

Neoplastic

Measles

Number of exacerbations during the year former :

Number of hospitalizations during the 2 years precedents:

Symptoms

Dyspnea effort : stadium mMRC /MRC

Hemoptysis : recurrent abundance

Cough : dry productive

Bronchorrhea morning

Pain thoracic : type

Recurrent lower respiratory infections

Spirometry

FEV (%)

FEV1/ FVC(%)

CVL (%)

ECBC

ATCD of Pseudomonas Aeruginosa infection : Colonization by Pseudomonas Aeruginosa Others germs : specify

---

Chest CT

Number of lobes:

Type of lesions:

Cylindrical / moniliforms / cystic
ADP: Mediastinal / hilars
Pleurisy
Emphysema

Quality of life assessment
Saint George questionnaire (SGRQ)

Etiology of the disease
Tuberculosis
Pneumonia at young age
System disease
Idiopathic
Others

Treatment
Inhaled corticosteroids
Corticosteroids systemic
Inhaled antibiotics
LAMA
OVER THERE
Theophylline
Bissolvan
Surgery : lobectomy / segmentectomy / pneumonectomy

Deaths / time between diagnosis and death

Severity scores **BSI score FACED score**

Annex 2: Charlson Comorbidity Index

Items	Weighting	Score
Myocardial infarction	1 point	
Insufficiency congestive heart	1 point	
Vascular diseases peripheral devices	1 point	
Cerebrovascular diseases (except hemiplegia)	1 point	
Dementia	1 point	
Lung diseases chronicles	1 point	
Tissue diseases connective	1 point	
Ulcers oeso -gastro- duodenal	1 point	
Uncomplicated diabetes	1 point	
Liver diseases light	1 point	
Hemiplegia	2 points	
Kidney diseases moderate Or severe	2 points	
Diabetes with impairment organ target	2 points	
Cancer	2 points	

Leukemia	2 points
Lymphoma	2 points
Multiple Myeloma	2 points
Disease hepatic moderate or severe	3 points
Tumor metastasized	6 points
AIDS	6 points

Annexe 3 : FACED score

Items	Points
Chronic colonisation by Pseudomonas Aeruginosa	
No	0
Yes	1
Dyspnoea mMRC score 0-II	0
III-IV	1
FEV1 % predicted	
>50%	0
<50%	2
Age	
<70 years	0
>70 years	2
Number of lobes 1-2	0
>2	1

Points	Score
0-2	Light DDB
3-4	Moderate DDB
5-7	Severe DDB

Annex 4: BSI score

Variable Points	
Age (year) <50	0
50-69	2
70-79	4
>80	6
Body mass index (BMI) <18.5	0
>18.5	2
FEV(%)	
>80%	0
50-80%	1

30-49%	2
<30%	3
Hospitalizations in the previous 2 years No	0
Yes	5
Exacerbations during the year previous 0-2	0
>3	2
Dyspnea - CKD 1-3	0
4	2
5	3
Colonization by Pseudomonas Aeruginosa No	0
Yes	3
Colonization by another microorganism No	0
Yes	1
Radiological extension (> 3 lobes and/ or cystic DDB)	0
No	1
Yes	

Points	Score
0-4	low BSI score
5-8	BSI score intermediate
> 9	BSI high score

Annex 5: HAD scale

Échelle HAD : *Hospital Anxiety and Depression scale*

L'échelle HAD est un instrument qui permet de dépister les troubles anxieux et dépressifs. Elle comporte 14 items cotés de 0 à 3. Sept questions se rapportent à l'anxiété (total A) et sept autres à la dimension dépressive (total D), permettant ainsi l'obtention de deux scores (note maximale de chaque score = 21).

1. Je me sens tendu(e) ou énervé(e)
- La plupart du temps 3
- Souvent 2
- De temps en temps 1
- Jamais 0

2. Je prends plaisir aux mêmes choses qu'autrefois
- Oui, tout autant 0
- Pas autant 1
- Un peu seulement 2
- Presque plus 3

3. J'ai une sensation de peur comme si quelque chose d'horrible allait m'arriver
- Oui, très nettement 3
- Oui, mais ce n'est pas trop grave 2
- Un peu, mais cela ne m'inquiète pas 1
- Pas du tout 0

4. Je ris facilement et vois le bon côté des choses
- Autant que par le passé 0
- Plus autant qu'avant 1
- Vraiment moins qu'avant 2
- Plus du tout 3

5. Je me fais du souci
- Très souvent 3
- Assez souvent 2
- Occasionnellement 1
- Très occasionnellement 0

6. Je suis de bonne humeur
- Jamais 3
- Rarement 2
- Assez souvent 1
- La plupart du temps 0

7. Je peux rester tranquillement assis(e) à ne rien faire et me sentir décontracté(e)
- Oui, quoi qu'il arrive 0
- Oui, en général 1
- Rarement 2
- Jamais 3

8. J'ai l'impression de fonctionner au ralenti
- Presque toujours 3
- Très souvent 2
- Parfois 1
- Jamais 0

9. J'éprouve des sensations de peur et j'ai l'estomac noué
- Jamais 0
- Parfois 1
- Assez souvent 2
- Très souvent 3

10. Je ne m'intéresse plus à mon apparence
- Plus du tout 3
- Je n'y accorde pas autant d'attention que je devrais 2
- Il se peut que je n'y fasse plus autant attention 1
- J'y prête autant d'attention que par le passé 0

11. J'ai la bougeotte et n'arrive pas à tenir en place
- Oui, c'est tout à fait le cas 3
- Un peu 2
- Pas tellement 1
- Pas du tout 0

12. Je me réjouis d'avance à l'idée de faire certaines choses
- Autant qu'avant 0
- Un peu moins qu'avant 1
- Bien moins qu'avant 2
- Presque jamais 3

13. J'éprouve des sensations soudaines de panique
- Vraiment très souvent 3
- Assez souvent 2
- Pas très souvent 1
- Jamais 0

14. Je peux prendre plaisir à un bon livre ou à une bonne émission de radio ou de télévision
- Souvent 0
- Parfois 1
- Rarement 2
- Très rarement 3

Scores

Additionnez les points des réponses : 1, 3, 5, 7, 9, 11, 13 : Total A = ______

Additionnez les points des réponses : 2, 4, 6, 8, 10, 12, 14 : Total D = ______

Interprétation

Pour dépister des symptomatologies anxieuses et dépressives, l'interprétation suivante peut être proposée pour chacun des scores (A et D) :

- 7 ou moins : absence de symptomatologie
- 8 à 10 : symptomatologie douteuse – 11 et plus : symptomatologie certaine.

Selon les résultats, il sera peut-être nécessaire de demander un avis spécialisé.

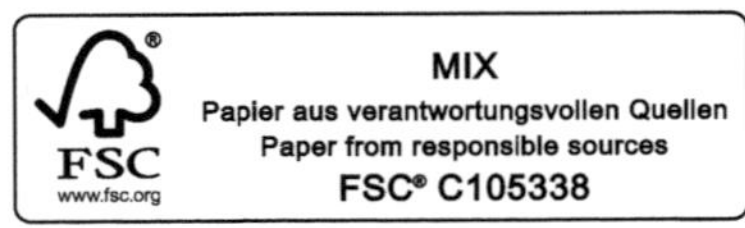

Printed by Books on Demand GmbH, Norderstedt / Germany